UNMASKING
CORONA

An approach to unveiling society's need to
accept shared responsibility

DERRICK H. SHORTRIDGE

WOW Book Publishing™

Dedication

Dedication

To my children, biological and non-biological... this is for your future.

Copyright

Copyright

First Edition Published by Derrick H. Shortridge

Copyright ©2021 Derrick H. Shortridge

WOW Book Publishing™

Testimonials

A well written account of what is a very topical issue – Unmasking Corona is a book for the public traversing education and societal discussions on not just the science of coronavirus but also the societal implications it has had.

It is a unique book in popular science that does not shy away from drawing parallels between biblical references and the current situation we are in.

This book offers the opportunity for a crash course in virology without ever attending a virology course/seminar. Perfect for those that want an insight into the conversations and complexity surrounding corona virus and what it tells us about the brokenness of society as we know it.

After reading this book a "business as usual approach" is no longer an option but should force us to act and make a change.

Dr. Riddick Owusu

(BSc, MBBS)

Testimonials

In this comprehensive, insightful and empirical text, Derrick Shortridge confronts, unveils and challenges the use, the abuse and the attention on masks, which has emerged on mass through and during the Covid pandemic which began in England in 2020. This book has been written to help us confront and take an honest look at the psychology of acceptance and resistance to the wearing of masks.

Its affect and effect on the environment and us all. I am blown away by his dedication to research and penmanship of such powerful words, where the reader can embrace the ease of access to such relevant, timely and thought-provoking information.

Information enmeshed in history, science and the present day, no-one is left doubting or without opinion. This book is a powerful and important contribution to the conversations surrounding masks, the pandemic, the environment and our own attitudes. The choice to be challenged or changed is yours and this book has the capacity to do both.

Michelle Campbell
Harmoni Counselling

Mr Shortridge was my secondary school science teacher and a force not to be reckoned with. Of all our teachers, he was one that always made ANY student come correct.

His reputation went before him in the school as a teacher not to mess about with, whether you were a student in his class or a student making noise in his corridor.

However, this reputation was based on students having the utmost respect for his time, teaching acumen and genuine father-like authority.

If you were on the end of a sharp reprimand by Mr Shortridge, you knew you would be impacted for life. He cared. Deep down, we all knew it and appreciated that his role as a teacher went far beyond the "periodic table".

"Unmasking Corona" challenges our preconceived ideas of the status quo in a manner where it is relatable and understandable to the reader, as a father would instruct and share with a child. Thank you for never losing that quality.

Dr Shadé Tongo (BSc, MBBS)

Acknowledgements

I want to thank my wife and children for believing in me. They were there in the dark and desperate years often sustaining me in ways I never knew I needed. Thanks to everyone on the WOW team who helped me so much. Special thanks to Pauline, the ever-patient Publishing Angel, and DJ, my amazing motivation.

To all my colleagues and friends, with whom I was educated, worked and played over the years, I appreciate you. I thank you for helping to shape me in so many ways.

Thank you to the Mico ... Squad 151, the entire batch, you are special. Including, but not exhaustive, Buck, Fredlocks, Chuck, Broadback, Teddy bear, CB, Tuckie, Roy, Bigboy ,Yellow Green and such... I have a heart filled with love for you all. To Angie, Rainess and the Home Economics option, you made my first birthday party – Mico would have never been the same without you...

The crew from my days at Happy Grove High school, my St. Ann massive, and my COP family much respect...

Finally, to Mr. R.G. Brown and the Browns family from Baillieston, my Trelawny friends and early teachers who together helped to mould me early. To my mother, father and grandmother dearly departed you all fostered my early development. All of my Shortridge family; my brothers, aunts, uncles, cousins, nieces and nephews much loved.

It is my prayer that all who read this book will be blessed by its contents and for you to tell your friends and family to read it as well.

Foreword

Dear Reader,

Unmasking Corona is the book you need to read and learn about to gain a perspective on how the pandemic has exposed some societal failings. It is a tool that makes it easier for us to get a real view on the lack of responsibility accepted by ordinary members of society.

Derrick has acquired some masterful skills and knowledge about the way society behaves. He has drawn attention to how People's behaviour is influenced by social norms: what they perceive that others are doing or what they think that others approve or disapprove of.

He has imparted it to you in a way that will allow you to understand and apply it immediately.

The knowledge in this book has the power to help you take stock of your life and how understanding and using guidance given by the powers that be with confidence.

X

I can tell you that even with my experience as successful author and international acclaimed speaker; I was amazed at his passion for the health of the world when I met him at the WOW BOOK CAMP.

Derrick has the drive, heart and is developing expertise to become a successful author. I am pleased with his progress as an author.

Vishal Mojaria
Award Winning Author
and International Speaker.

Table of Contents

Prologue

Unmasking Corona is a book about buried truths unveiled by the pandemic sweeping around the globe. More specifically, it is a book on what we know and how that knowledge informs our ability to make responsible decisions. I used the Bible to reference many of the points I explore, marrying scriptural references to modern-day reality. We need to be well-grounded in the subject. The biblical teaching about responsibility is understudied and grossly misunderstood. While writing this book and recounting some events, I cringed, verged on tears, and grappled with the rollercoaster of emotions.

During the year of the first major global pandemic, I noticed some home truths that inspired me to pick up my pen. Writing is something I was encouraged to do for many, many years. In 2003 whilst I was transcribing the interviews for one of my theses, Mr. R.G. Brown (my first mentor who was holidaying in England with his wife, Angela and whilst spending a few days with me) remarked to the following effect. "So, Derrick, you are working hard on this man. Why don't you write your memoirs? I think you should write your memoirs; there is a lot you could say."

We had just returned from a day out in London, viewing the city from the London Eye, and checking out the city when the remark was made. The statement kept me thinking for years, but I did little if anything about it.

Prologue

I never dreamed that a pandemic would be the catalyst that woke me from that slumber and caused me to burst into action. With the foundation established some seventeen years before, my eldest child completed her master's degree in Pharmacy; my middle boy was in his second year at University studying for a degree in Criminology with an eye on Forensics. It was one morning as I walked my youngest son along the route he would be taking to school as he embarked on his final year in primary school that it hit me. Etched in my mind was the picture of a dog-tired nurse making a tearful impassioned plea to the British public to refrain from panic-buying. She returned home after completing a grueling 48-hours shift to find supermarket shelves empty.

Having observed many, many masks discarded in several different and exciting places, my phone came out, and the idea of taking photographs was born. I discussed with DJ the prospect of doing a project to educate the populace on the dangers of litter and especially masks since it had become mandatory to wear them in buildings in the UK. It was excellent speaking to my son, who had an appetite for a good conversation and kept me thinking at a level that belied his years. This ten-year-old knew more about Pythagoras and the stegosaurus than I will ever know.

I knew first-hand because of my interactions with young people and their parents during my tenure as a science teacher and head of the secondary school department. The enforcement of the mask-wearing would prove difficult. Over time spent in public life, I saw fifteen years of decay, cracks, and fissures in society's fabric. It was apparent to me that morality in the community; British society was not in free fall but was at the bottom of the fall. It hit with a great thud; the gravity of entitlement carried the mass of racism, lawlessness, and protests brought it down at supersonic speed. In the west, American, Europe and UK society, anything goes. Religious beliefs, especially Islam and Christianity, are breeding grounds.

Jack from Camden, a medical doctor on the frontline, poured his heart out about me, me, me culture they are continually thinking about their own needs. He pointed out that the conversation heard on some fronts may about "I will not die from COVID-19"; he said that they may not die from that disease but will die from leukaemia diabetes and heart disease... "Every person who gets sick with the disease does so from contact with another person earlier". We will call him Dr Jack from here, and he said the nurses in the NHS are the lifeblood of the service but they not valued. This caller to LBC, a London-based radon station mentioned having evidence that compassion and personal responsibility worked. He identified illegal music events and other selfish undertakings as leading to increased death rates.

In politics, good manners and tolerance of other people's viewpoints have all but evaporated. Governments behaved despicably in the discharge of their duties; dishonesty, nepotism and outright corruption are commonplace. I saw earnings declining, businesses going bust, race relations decaying, factions planning unrests, and national debts skyrocketing. We are not safe in our world anymore; the pandemic has exposed the underbelly of a deadly serpent. The world is unstable, seen in ways many of us have never seen in our lifetimes, leading to mass insecurity and anxiety. Our leaders show impotence in discharging their duties on all fronts, from global to regional to local, where targets are continually moving and the onset of a worldwide pandemic. If we listen to the dissemination of information from the UK government, for example, they have been behind the pinball all the way through, one caller to a radio show made it clear[2].

Vaccine rollouts are not straight forward, and as such, the powers that be have to be 'fleet of foot', displaying agility as circumstances change. With the public disconnected from scientific truths because of many reasons, a vacuum is left in their knowledge base. This space gets filled with 'vlogs' about sensational events; many containing only half truths. From these posts they receive gratification in monetary terms, 'subscriptions', 'likes' and 'shares'.

I believe we have turned away from the most outstanding support available; God relegated and replaced by allies who have no compassion; countries were fighting to break up age-old unions and no longer trust each other. One commentator remarked that '… our other allies do not trust us; our enemies no longer fear us, and the world no longer respects us[1]'. It became clear to many people that ominous clouds were gathering, and many are asking, "Is this the end? [3]" – Dr David Jeremiah was speaking about America.

Instead of taking responsibility, it appears that excuses are the default position of so many in our world. Many of the population would agree with my summation that the culture, economics, belief systems, morality, and civility are mired in a critical state of deterioration never seen before. Fear and anxiety engulf the people with from all classes, creeds, races, vocations, and professions with whom I speak. As I acknowledge that things cannot go on the way they are for much longer and along came the COVID-19 pandemic.

The world is asking if we are in the last throes of life as we know it. Both Christians and secularists wonder if this is what the Bible taught; records show that internet searches for bible references about what is playing out before our eyes have increased massively in the recent past. Schools, Brexit, elections and health became pawns used to play the game of 'whodunit' in Britain while the west (America) and the east (China) battle over the rights for the conception of a pandemic like no one has ever seen for a century.

Secularists are asking if the disorder playing out is down to what Christians call the Rapture (the belief that all dead and living believers will ascend to heaven at the second coming). Church folks are wavering and wondering if we see Revelation (the end times according to scripture) unfolding. Is it a case of economic, ethnic, cultural, and political chaos on the cusp of descent? Whether the millennial generation is imploding or whether a hostile nation like Iran, China, or Russia might unleash 'cyberfury' on our governments. Or if, as the scripture promised, plagues would breach our borders and inflict sufficient harm to bring us to our knees.

The anxiety is not unprecedented; the tale about the London Nazi blitz began in late 1940. Londoners quickly set an emergency system of air-raid sirens and bomb shelters.

Prologue

Children back then were carted off to the countryside and to other safe towns. The scenes at the time were not dissimilar to what we see now; before they were evacuated the children and adults faced disorganisation, terrifying screams of falling bombs, the roar of planes overhead and gunfire from aircraft guns as bombs exploded on the city of London[4]. The world seems to be collapsing; superpowers of the UK, America, Russia, and an emerging China continue to look for dominance in the theatre. As the climate changes, we wonder if there is any responsibility in the world while pondering if there is any sanctuary place.

We are confident that things cannot continue the way they are, so we wonder, is there an end to this madness? 'Corona' has been blamed for where we are as a world; we ask ourselves if it is the end of time. What is clear is that we are watching a planet in crisis un-boxing what seems to be a catalogue of disasters; fires, floods and famine appear to be commonplace. While the world sleepwalks into chaos the systemic essence of it allows the shunning of accountability.

The unfolding chapters here will address these questions seeking to unmask controversies and inequalities in our society. I will attempt to avoid over-promising by quickly saying that some of the answers we are looking for remain masked by the façade, and only the mind of God can reveal them. Only God knows our fate will be given the scope of the problems we face as a people.

My answer to the question about to the question of hope is; "Yes! There is still hope – a cherished desire for change for the better to come. Behind the mask is a reality that God is real and controls the earth outside of time and space eternally. We must make sure though, that we do not misplace the Hope of which I speak. We have seen the world written off before, areas of the Middle East, the Far East, America, and Britain have seen revolutions through the years.

There have been two world wars, Spanish flu pandemics, Tsunamis, and earthquakes throughout history. But in each event, the nations survived the crisis and surged forward with improved strength and energy. Incidents of Governments using the plight of nations as political footballs are evident in western society where mixed messages pour out of different quarters frequently.

The question about revival remains after the latest episode in history. Whether or not we will be able to strip off the mask covering our descent into instability and lack of humanity still begs. It might or it might not; we should not concern ourselves with whether we will regain stability, or if we are hoping against Hope. It is about whether all of us worldwide will take responsibility and respond as a collective to the unfolding issues. This book seeks to explore these and other issues.

When I interact with people in my life; from school, church or shops, there are some common responses to the growing fears about our world's future. The first response that I get and abhor is denial; many people are doing the 'ostrich', with their heads firmly buried in the sand. I see them living on the illusion that the SARS-CoV-2 virus is not real and that all the factors around it, like masks, social distancing, and vaccination will not change anything. The storm clouds gathering over the horizon not taken seriously. Another ominous sign behind the mask is despair; breakdown will come, all is lost, schools closed, business going under and hopelessness abounds.

They say we can do nothing, and we are a doomed people. Our hearts have filled with terror that is induced by sorrow and despair. People are worried sick about death, which results in hordes of them cramming in as many pleasures as possible, just crossing off many things from their bucket list "because a man has nothing better under the sun than to eat drink and be merry."[5] There is nothing constructive in any of these answers since none offers any hope behind the mask.

People reaching out to me say, "I am scared" or "I am surprised at the level of my anxiety". In all honesty, many of us have experienced worrying moments, some qualms in one form or other. Right at the minute, most have something to lose such as health, home finances, jobs and forgotten groups of self-employed people in Britain not having worked for months on end without government support... Future looking shrouded in darkness.

The silver lining is behind these dark clouds, this issue behind the mask – Hope is a reliable platform; God himself offers Hope. There is Hope in the future of the world, and stability is but a fleeting wish. It is unreliable. The Hope God provides - the only realistic, absolute Hope that conveys the promise of a positive result. The end of the world will not come to an end immediately, according to bible scholars. No one knows when the Lord will return.

Hope is one of many people's favourite words; it is a promise, a confident expression that all things will work out for us. It is a full guarantee of a positive future. As we navigate this pandemic, it is apparent that people are losing hope because of the presence of inept governance, and the outcome of the next year was a mystery.

We need to remember that our souls' enemy wants to kill, steal, and destroy.[6] Our Hope is a bounty for him but we have that assurance from the Word that we have a great future in God. Our Hope should be a beacon in this dark world, and we need to start by establishing Hope in our homes.

Joy[7], love[8], boldness[9], and perseverance[10]; the foundation of our Hope is the grace of God[11]: "*Now may our Lord Jesus Christ himself, and God our Father, who loved us and gave us eternal comfort and good hope through grace, comfort your hearts and establish them in every good work and word*"[12]

Behind the mask is the face that has etched on it despair, worry, fear, anxiety, and other raw emotions. God's desire is for us to live without the desire to control the future, and that is why we become anxious. The Bible lists many cases of hopelessness turning to Hope. Borne out by the fact according to scripture that God offers you "thoughts of peace and not evil", and he desires us to have "a future of hope"[13].

9

Chapter 1

Viral diseases are commonplace...
It's not all about COVID-19.

Education for basic understanding

Infectious diseases have been around a long time. The microorganisms that cause these diseases are usually classified as pathogens and commonly called germs[1]. Infections are more likely to occur if larger numbers of germs enter the body due to poor hygienic conditions or contact with infected animals, people, or surfaces.

These germs make you feel ill by causing damage to body tissues and by producing toxins (poisons) which cause you to feel symptoms and see signs to effects including high temperature, nausea, headache, diarrhea and vomiting[1].

The feelings do not appear immediately after infection and can take different periods from hours to days. The period from infection to experiencing symptoms or displaying signs is called the incubation period, during which time the germs multiply swiftly inside your body[2].

Viruses are one group of pathogens that are problematic because of their size and nature. Virology is the scientific discipline within the biological sciences that involves the study of viruses[3]. I know the Creation biologists study viruses, and creationists have published numerous papers on this subject. They are not cells and are unable to exist without the aid of a host cell for very long, and as a result, we refer to them as the ultimate parasites.

This means they use the host's partition for their benefit by using its biochemistry while causing the host to suffer harm[4]. Unlike living organisms, viruses do not carry out all the vital functions of life. They do not feed, grow, move autonomously, or respire. They use the body's systems to get around. Viruses produce proteins, called movement proteins, to overcome the organism's control of the cells. Viruses hijack cells and turn them into mini factories.

The virus that causes COVID-19 is very robust; it is a lipid-enveloped virus surrounded by RNA[5]. This means it is covered in fat. I will mention more about this later in this chapter and in proceeding chapters but at this point it should be noted that there are at least six types of corona viruses that can cause considerable diseases to humans[6].

How does Severe Acute Respiratory Syndrome [SARS-CoV-2] cause disease?

The corona virus enters through the nose or mouth, and can spread via surfaces, but the jury is still out on how long it can stay on them. Droplet transmission seems to be the primary way of spreading the virus. When people cough or sneeze, you

touch a person who is ill or by rubbing your eyes, nose or touching your face - Hands! Face! Space! - British slogan.[1]
From here, it awaits an opportunity to thumb a ride to its destination, which is the intestines, lungs, or spleen.

These organs provide the most fertile ground for the virus to set up shop and deploy their troops into the body. Just for clarity, COVID-19 is not a new virus as so many ill informed politicians, bureaucrats, technocrats and autocrats spout on a daily basis. It is actually the name in which the disease caused by a new virus in the corona virus family of viruses. Other diseases that are similar in nature are SARS (Severe Acute Respiratory Syndrome) and MERS-CoV (Middle East Respiratory Syndrome)[3] first discovered in Saudi Arabia in 2012.

It was predicted early in the pandemic that, SARS-CoV-2 has two main virulence factors which cause illness. The first is known as, nsp-1, and it restrains the early warning immune system factor called *interferon* (A protein produced by cells in response to virus infection that inhibits viral replication)[4]. The second is called "S" factor and activates immune system messengers that heighten the readiness of the immune system. Having both these factors active in COVID-19 provides the ideal basis for intensifying disease.

The virus is then able to bypass the early warning immune system and can trigger inflammation to extremely high levels[5]. The most devastating effect on the lungs is that it damages the epithelium [covering cells that line our bodies' surfaces] and are a prime area for infection – a weak point in the perimeter in war parlance. They contain DNA (Deoxyribonucleic Acid), or RNA (ribonucleic acid) protein encased in an envelope of fat. These are the largest of all RNA – containing viruses.

They attach themselves to the cell membrane by connecting to a receptor on the surface of the cells - fits it perfectly like a hand in a glove (The biologists among us know what this is about.) The outer spike protein of the virus latches on to specific receptors on the surface of cells – in the case of SARS-CoV-2 it latches on to the ac2 receptors and this marks the beginning of the process where the virus fuses into human cells[6]. They then inject their DNA into the cytoplasm of the cell where chemical reactions take place.

Genetically the blueprint of the virus is RNA which instructs the host cell machinery to read the instructions and translate it into protein that make up new virus particles. Note this is not the DNA that many misinformers spout; the cell is now taken 'prisoner' and executes their instructions which are simple to copy and reassemble mitosis. Once it uses the DNA of the host cell continues to make more copies of the virus, assemble them into workable particles and move them to the edges of the cell before release.

Each infected cell release hundreds of clones of itself being able to infect neighbouring cells and people when they are expelled through the airways by coughing and sneezing in droplets. The virus then issues one final order: to self-destruct; in as little as half an hour, the host cell bursts, and the new

13

virus clones are released to infect other cells in the host organism. After several days, in SARS-CoV-2, the current novel corona virus, millions of body cells are infected, and billions of viruses have produced, and the invasion is complete. At this point, your body becomes its own worst enemy, the signaling system hijacked, and the messaging is now in the control of the enemy.

The immune system, now on instruction, attacks the invaders; the response is automatic. The cells (soldiers) then get deployed to fight the virus (invaders) and pour into the cells in an all-out attack. Because of the lack of coordination by the communication command, the messaging is chaotic. Because cells do not have organs, so no ears or eyes; their communication uses cytokines. These control nearly every significant immune reaction.

Now what happens to you is critical; the immune response at this point is to send many more (cells) 'soldiers' to the site than is necessary putting them into turmoil and causing serious damage. I see two types of cells here causing pandemonium; first, some *Neutrophils* are killing everything in sight, including good cells as they arrive in their thousands.

As if that is not enough, the second company is known as Killer T-CELLS that, in normal circumstances, order infected cells to commit suicide. However, because of the state of confusion, they instruct healthy cells to do the same... owing to the vast numbers of cells that are dying, the lung tissue dies off.

Reports are that this can get so bad that irreversible damage results and the person has difficulty breathing since the alveoli became permanently scarred. This can lead to potential lifelong disabilities, one example is 'long COVID' an emerging problem from this pandemic.

In most instances, the battle goes on for a while. Eventually, the cytokines regain control of the messaging and kill the infected cells, intercepts the viruses trying to invade healthy cells and cleans up the frontline. This process is the start of the recovery, so rest and good nutrition are now paramount. Most people infected with corona will usually recover with relatively mild symptoms; a dry cough, sneeze, or loss of taste, but we do not know the exact percentages because of the fluid nature of the disease caused by the novel corona virus.

What we know is that there are more critical cases than with the flu. With COVID-19, the acute instances show that a more significant portion of the lung's epithelial lining gets damaged. The alveoli that are usually robust and resistant to bacterial infection get compromised, giving rise to pneumonia where respiration becomes hard. Respiration is the transfer of energy from nutrients; usually, glucose burnt in oxygen.

To obtain the oxygen; gases get exchanged between the lungs and the bloodstream. Whenever this occurs, there is reduced uptake of this important gas and the body functions at a much-reduced capacity. The patient requires ventilation at this point because the alveoli are unable to get air in and out automatically. The immune system has fought now for weeks at full tilt and produced millions of antiviral weapons.

15

However, now the body is faced with a bacterial infection, and these antivirals cannot fight bacteria. Your body now requires antibodies to be produced, but it is overwhelmed by depletion in resources and energy. Hence, bacteria enter the bloodstream and besiege the body, leading to death in many instances.

Typical examples are corona viruses, so named because of their crown shape with the protein jolting out from the surface. There are about six types that are known to cause disease to humans. Influenza, (flu) the highly contagious, acute viral infection of the respiratory tract, has been around forever and a day and affects millions of people annually.

Comparisons of the COV1D-19 virus and the flu show similarities, but we know that it is much more contagious (infectious) and spreads much faster than the flu. We have learnt to live with it taking precautions where possible. Other viral diseases include polio and smallpox (practically eliminated), Ebola, Measles, Mumps, Rubella, and Yellow fever.

Vaccine Efficacy explained

Safety and efficacy around the dosage of vaccines is an issue... the clarity and strength of information from the vaccines need to come to the forefront so you can allay vaccine phobia - Joint Committee on Vaccination and Immunisation (JCVI); 50% or more protection from vaccines is excellent. If people realise the vaccination is only part of the armoury of tools for fighting the infections it might assist them in fight…

Responsibility… Deputy chair of JCVI said GPs are under tremendous pressure and fight back regarding the rollout time scale for the vaccine programme. The importance of this is that the vaccine would get into it into as many people as possible as quickly as possible… new strains are the is the issue, the Brazilian, Kent, South African and most recently the Indian variants are in the public consciousness. The research findings reported in different parts of the world by scientists and media houses described the viruses using codes that led to confusion. In a move to squash the confusion that led to geographical stigmas it was agreed that the strains would be named with Greek letters.

To date the designation is as Alpha – Dec 2020, Beta – Dec 2020, Gamma - Jan 2021, Delta – May 2021[1]. This system served to help convey clearer information according to Jeffery Barrett. The statistical geneticist leading SARS-CoV-2 sequencing efforts at the Wellcome Sanger Institute in Hinxton, UK opined."It is a lot easier for a radio newsreader to say 'Delta' than B.1.617.2; so I'm willing to give it a try to help it 'take off'"[2]

"Let's hope it sticks," says Tulio de Oliveira, a bioinformatician and director of the kwaZulu- Natal Research Innovation and sequencing and Sequencing Platform in Durban, South Africa, whose team identified the Beta variant. "I find the names quite simple and easy"[3]

Many are fooled using technical language and end up with misinformation overload. The arguments and counter arguments about vaccines and their efficacy are no different. When referred to in the context of the ongoing pandemic it means that the percentage number simply tells how the vaccine performed in clinical trials; there is no way of predicting the performance of the vaccines in the real world. The view of many experts is that efficacy is not the best measure of how good a vaccine is anyway. It should be the aim of governments and health authorities to tame the virus, to take its 'sting' away by removing its ability to cause illness, hospitalisation and death in society.

When politicians attempt to make a case for the use of vaccine from a position of ignorance it is no wonder, we see instances like in the case of the mayor of Detroit city in USA. He was to receive more than 6000 doses of the vaccine developed by Johnson and Johnson; the single dose vaccine with an efficacy 66%. He promptly declined the shipment claiming he want the people of his city to get 'only the best'. Mr. Mayor claimed Moderna and Pfizer BioNTech were the best, having 94% and 95% efficacy rate respectively. The Sputnik V vaccine from Russia (92%), Novax (89%) and Oxford/Astra Zeneca (67%) completed the suite of vaccine available now[4].

The efficacy numbers are arguably not even the most important in the grand scheme of understanding how effective the vaccines are and a good knowledge of what vaccine are supposed to do is essential. The efficacy rates are calculated from data collected in large trials; tests are done on tens of thousands of people[5]. They are put into two groups with half getting the vaccine and the other half getting a placebo (a harmless substance like the vaccine that contains no active ingredients) then they are both sent away to live normally for a prescribed period, usually several months, while scientists monitor them. The results would then be analysed and information about how many people contracted the disease would give the vaccine efficacy[6].

If the number of infected people in the trial is spread evenly between the two groups it would mean one is just as likely to get the disease with the vaccine as without it, so it would have a zero percent efficacy. On the other hand, if all the infected persons were from the group that was given the placebo, then the vaccine would have 100% efficacy. In the trial of 43000 people that Pfizer Bio N Tech undertook 162 persons out of the 170 infected were in the placebo group meaning only 8 persons (5%) in the group with the COVID-19 vaccine got the infection.

Even though 95% of the persons fell into the placebo group it doesn't mean that 95 out of every 100 persons were protected from the infection. Instead, it referred to an individual with the vaccine is 95% less likely to get the infection each time they are exposed to the virus than a person who has not been vaccinated. We should note that every vaccine's efficacy rate is calculated in the same manner, but each trial might be done in vastly different circumstances.

In the case of the COVID-19, one of the biggest factors when looking at the efficacy numbers is the timing in which the clinical trials were performed. A snapshot of the number of daily cases in the United States since the start of the COVID-19 pandemic began showed that the Moderna trial was done entirely in the USA in the summer of 2020 and the Pfizer BioNtech also mainly based there as well.

Critically, however, the Johnson and Johnson vaccine trials were done later and at the peak of the pandemic when there was a greater likelihood that more participants would be more exposed to infection. Also, most of their trials took place in other parts of the world in places like South Africa, and Brazil where the case rates of the disease was not only high, but the virus was different.

The South African and Brazilian variants that were more likely to get participants ill emerged and dominated the populations. Johnson and Johnson found that in South Africa most of the cases in the trial were that of the variant and not of the original virus strain which appeared in the USA over the summer and the vaccine performed well in preventing infections.

To test the vaccines in a head-to-head would not be fair because they were not trialled at the same time with the same controls in the same parts of the globe and inclusion criteria. It is safe to say that if the Pfizer BioNtech, Moderna, Oxford/ Astra Zeneca, Sputnik V, Novax with Johnson, and Johnson at the same time we might see different results entirely. It is important to note that through all the trials people in the placebo groups were taken ill, hospitalised and some even died. However, not even one participant in the vaccinated groups was hospitalised or died from COVID-19.

The Detroit mayor and many like him that go around making invalidated statements about vaccination should take time to learn. They can be assured that the science proved that the vaccine from whichever one of the providers is 100% capable of protecting the population dying from the virus. As one researcher put it "The best vaccine you can get right now it the one you are offered." There are so many corners of the word without access to vaccines.

What do we do in this pandemic...?

Pandemics have two outlooks fast or slow, much depends on how we approach them when they start. Corona virus Disease 2019 (COVID-19) [coronavirus] is a fast pandemic; the history books will record costing many lives, way over one million people have died so far, around eighteen months into it. Much depends on how we react to pandemics; if numbers of infected people get too large, health care systems become overwhelmed and unable to handle it. Resources become scarce; health care staff gets ill and horrible decision must be made about the deployment of resources; who gets to live and who dies...

The world must take collective responsibility for reducing this COV-19 to a slow pandemic by enacting the right responses primarily because, in some sectors of society, the early phase response was less than adequate.

Since there was no fully authorised vaccine for COVID-19 and that they are available, we had to and need to engineer our behaviour to act like a social vaccine. To do this, we must do a few things, firstly try our hardest not to get infected. And to realize this, we must follow reasonable guidelines from the experts and of conscience. The second is crucial and probably more contentious; not infecting others. Although it sounds trivial, washing of hands is critical in stopping infection, soap is a powerful tool here since the corona virus is encased in a layer of fat. The simple explanation is that soap breaks down the fat, and the virus gets destroyed and washed away.

Scripture says "In this, you greatly rejoice, though now for a little while, if need be, you have been grieved by various trials, that the genuineness of your faith, being much more precious than gold that perishes, though tested by fire, may be found to praise, honour, and glory at the revelation of Jesus Christ, who having not seen you love[1]."

Viral diseases spread from person to person by several means; from direct contact through handshakes and cuddles to touching objects such as doorknobs, coins, and books. Touching the nose, mouth or face are easy ways of contracting the virus. Hand washing must be a way of life going forward; it must be frequent and thorough using soap and warm water; as it dissolves the virus's fatty protein coating[2].

Animal vectors also spread diseases; mosquitoes are a notorious one that spreads deadly viruses[3]. Yellow fever is one example of a disease caused by a virus that damages the victim's liver. Corona viruses are present in many animals and have caused many conditions throughout the decades, including bird flu, swine flu and SARS[4]. Another case in point turns out to be the global pandemic gripping the world now caused by the SARS-CoV-2 novel corona virus. It is linked to bats in wet markets in China and minks in Denmark more recently[5].

The SARS-CoV-2 virus that causes COVID-19 gripped and hugged the headlines since the turn of the year 2020. When it did it masked the fact and took the spotlight off AIDS and Influenza that are still are still around and killing thousands. To date America had reported around 32.26 million cases with around 617,000 dead from COVID-19 at the time of writing. Soon we will enter another winter season where influenza will be killing people again[6]. Of the over 206,254,882 million patients of COVID-19 worldwide - Statista and the New Times reports at the time of writing, one million people died.

In six American states, another real threat of another mosquito-borne infection by the virus known as "Triple E" (Eastern Equine Encephalitis) was rampant. ABC News in the USA reported that the crisis unfolded in the state of Massachusetts where a woman died on Sunday, September 27, 2020.

Patients could go from being perfectly normal to paralyzed or even dead within 24 to 48 hrs, a point made by Dr Todd Ellerin. Communities need to be spraying and making sure the breeding sites for mosquitoes no longer exist.

My instinct was and still is that we could dwell on these numbers and enter a Zombie state where we get to toss on the seas of uncertainty and disillusion by the deluge of news from both mainstream and social media[7]. David Phillips spoke (*The magical science of storytelling | David JP Phillips | TEDX Stockholm)* recently about the hormones in our bodies and how the body copes. Our levels of cortisol (the naturally occurring pregnane corticosteroid and is also known as 11β, 17α, 21-trihydroxypregn-4-ene-3, 20-Dione) and adrenaline rise because the situation is terrifying and nerve-racking. The increased agitation experienced by the populace, especially the very elderly and young adults, makes for gross intolerance, high irritability, criticism, and, most detrimental, a lack of creativity.

A nugget of hope was information gleaned from NHS data available at the time was as follows, *'COVID-19 is a new illness that can affect your lungs and airways. It is caused by a virus called SAR-COV- 2.*

The 'coronavirus'' (COVID-19) main symptoms are a high temperature, a new, continuous cough, and a loss or change to your sense of smell or taste.

To help stop the spread of coronavirus (COVID-19), avoid close contact with anyone you do not live with and regularly wash your hands.

You can usually treat mild coronavirus (COVID-19) symptoms at home. If your symptoms are severe, you may need medical care until you recover'.

Pharmacy vigilance is essential because several thoughts need exploration for us to better understand the facts around how to adapt in this pandemic[8]. It is extremely critical since vaccination is one of the most important interventions for the prevention of illness or at least the reduction in the need for hospitalisation in emergency circumstances as is the case with the global COVID-19 pandemic.

Like other pharmaceutical products, vaccines are not completely free from perils and things happen that have adverse effects ranging from minor side effects to more severe responses[9]. It is noteworthy that the general tolerance and acceptance of events following was low and, in some contexts, could he still low mainly because vaccines are usually given to healthy people to prevent the onset of disease. This therefore requires a higher safety standard for immunisations in comparison to other treatment modes.

The SAR-CoV-2 is one of several corona viruses, and viruses mutate by nature in order to survive. One of the mutations at earlier in the pandemic showed in the mink population in Denmark. At around June 2020, it was revealed that minks could pass on corona virus to humans. Due to a mutation in the virus, maybe 12 people had been infected with the virus strain. Probably the full impact will be known when the world's population returned to a lockdown; there have been a fair few.

The area in Denmark where cases were identified went into lockdown immediately after. These animals were culled, and it is estimated that around 17 million across hundreds of mink-producing farms produced these for the fur lucrative markets. Matt Hancock in Britain addressed Parliament on how the UK responded to the news. He banned travel from Denmark and ordered isolation of 14 days for those returning home from that country. Testing became a big part of the fight against the virus and the lateral flow test, which is also called as immune chromatographic, assays[10] or rapid tests turned around in 15 minutes being available to most of the UK population where Liverpool and Stoke and Trent were two of the areas where it was most widely used...

I noted with interest that this small Scandinavian country's premier had indicated that the SAR– CoV-2 viruses that cause COVID -19 could spread in minks. Wait a minute; this is the virus we knew transferred from bats or snakes in Wuhan China. What is going on here? The strains in minks are finding themselves around the world and in people...

It spread across Europe; different parts of the continent were experiencing outbreaks[11], a point postulated by Emma Hodcroft (dubbed 'the virus hunter' in the trade), and geneticist at the University of Basel in Switzerland. Her field of study was the changing nature of corona viruses. There were those waiting for the study exponent to reveal the genetic code of the modified strain. She co-authored a piece with Adam S. Lauring MD, PhD for the JAMA Network where they explained mutations, variants and the spread in an easy to understand style. Interestingly and perfect for a point I will later make they pointed out that mutations in corona viruses were much less than other RNA viruses because they encode a particular enzyme that corrects some of the errors that lead to mutations.[12].

The influenza virus has a vaccine, and the efficacy is around 40%. I noted with interest that the seasonal inoculation of flu vaccines obviated the doctors' visits, hospitalisation, and deaths in the west over the years. Much of this work done on the back of estimations based on the season before the forthcoming season. It was not possible to have the vaccine for the current season as the previous virus could have mutated.

It intrigues me that this can be an acceptable course of action since viruses are specific [with peculiar structures] and are named A, B, C and D. We know the Human Influenza A and B viruses cause seasonal flu epidemics[13]. A significant number of countries experience seasonal flu every autumn/winter and the respiratory symptoms may be more serious and can lead to complications like triggering asthma attacks.

The 'S' [or spike] proteins that plays a pivotal role in penetrating the host and beginning the infection of cells on invasion is present on the surface of viruses[14] … it stays there even if the virus is dead…

RNA vaccine consists of a section of the genetic code of the virus; an instruction manual for the SARS-CoV-2. The immune response will produce the T- cells that will identify the virus and be ready to attack it[15]. (The scouse scientist – Professor Tom Solomon from the University of Liverpool.)

Epidemics of old include bird flu (H5N1 since 1997) and AIDS was caused by evolving viruses. At the turn of the decade of the 90s, there were several emerging viruses. Studies have focused on the interaction of viruses with hosts and the continued study of microbes, making it easier to track behaviour of new ones. As the nineties meandered into the noughties, SARS came into focus. China also appeared in the consciousness of the world; the barrier between species was breached. Viruses jumped from animals to humans and spread along the trails forged by increased air transportation in our global economy. SARS spread to over thirty countries on literally all continents. Science came to the rescue as it usually does. SARS in 2003 that originated in Asia was halted by synergy between countries never seen before. The virus showed how exposed humans were to infectious diseases. The previous two decades saw the rapid spread of contagious diseases and SARS outbreaks we should have seen from the research. This was a signal that the world would continue to see the emergence of new viral infections.

Different influenza strains, from the Spanish flu of 1918 to H1N1 (swine flu) in 2009 caused a pandemic and in 2019 SARS-CoV-2 found to cause COVID-19 becoming another of these cross-species viruses.

Be educated… get vaccinated.

The human body can naturally use active immunity to prevent and cure infections. Vaccination exploits our ability to acquire active immunity.

A vaccine is a preparation of a disease-causing agent, its components, or its products to induce active immunity.

Modern medicine relies heavily on the exploitation and stimulation of the natural process of active immunity. The WHO points out that each pathogen is made up of multiple subparts that are usually exclusive to that particular pathogen and the disease it causes. The subparts enable the production of antibodies (technically called antigens[1].) The production of vaccines (containing antigens) which stimulate the adaptive immune response was first pioneered by an English country doctor called Edward Jenner in 1756.

In the late 18th century, smallpox was a much-feared disease; it was called the 'speckled monster' due to its distinctive blister-like rashes, and it had killed millions since primitive times[2].

When a smallpox epidemic hit his home county of Gloucestershire in 1788, Jenner made several important observations about the disease. At which point, the records show that this was largest cause of death in Europe; killing in the region of 400,000 every year at the time[3]. A team of researchers hunted the virus, sequenced its genetic code, and then recreated it in a safe laboratory environment. It was this time that the CDC was set up in the USA to unearth the secrets of the virus and prepare for future pandemics[4].

Jenner observed that milkmaids and others who encountered cattle rarely suffered from smallpox. He also noticed that these workers faced cowpox (a disease related to smallpox, but much less virulent). Jenner theorised that the pus in the blisters which the milkmaids developed from cowpox protected them from smallpox. Some people felt then that using the cowpox was unhealthy and medicine had not evolved to the levels we experience today. In May 1796, Jenner tested his theory by inoculating the young James Phipps with material extracted from the cowpox sores found on the hand of the milkmaid

Sarah Nelmes. James Phipps became ill with the cowpox and, several weeks later, Jenner injected him with material containing the smallpox virus [Jenner also vaccinated his son - as shown in the statue erected in his memory.] James Phipps survived and did not suffer from smallpox.

The 'the father of immunology', Jenner, concluded that infection with cowpox provided immunity to smallpox, and he laid the foundations for the practice of vaccination, a method that is safe and ethical when carried out properly. We now know that this happened because the cowpox and smallpox viruses have a similar antigen, and therefore the acquired immunity worked against both diseases. Corona viruses are a family, just as there are Poxviruses causing chickenpox, smallpox, and cowpox.

Jenner's work was met with much skepticism and ridicule at first. However, following further work and technique improvement, Jenner's discovery was eventually accepted, and in 1840 smallpox vaccination was provided to the British population free of charge[5]. That was not the end of that, also immediately there were banners bearing the slogan "Repeal the Vaccinations Acts, the curse of our nation" and pledging "Better a felon's cell than a poisoned babe." In this era vaccination was vilified; the smallpox was a gruesome affair[6]. I wonder if what is happening now is a replay of this chapter in history.

Inoculation required them to have deep cuts in their arms and the material from a previously infected child put into it. The old approach to medicine made these open wounds vulnerable to gangrene, blood poisoning and other infections. It was not uncommon to see the burning of the hated laws in the streets. The humble country doctor's effigy hanging in the wind has been the programme's architect promoting smallpox prevention. Later on the media of the day, Royal Cornwall Gazette from December 1886 stated: **'Some of these poor infants have been borne of pillows for weeks, decaying alive before death ended their sufferings'[7].**

Today we have social media spewing disinformation into the voids created by lack of clarity of thought from the world's leaders. People without information react to what is available to them and get labeled *'anti-vaxxers'*. In Jenner's day, the opposition to vaccination was met with very prompt and extremely vicious cartoons depicting the vaccines as cow-like monsters feasting on children. Reportedly "This came from various angles, for example, sanitation, religious, scientific and political."[8] - (Dr Kristin Hussey). It is important to note that although the world has been rid of the dreaded smallpox virus for many years, doubters are still around.

Some people refused to accept that transmission of smallpox was from person to person while others just refused to be told what to do or what was right for them. This is a sentiment shared by too many in our modern adult society. It is bad enough to stumble in the dark, but the world casts off the knowledge of God, lacking restraint and guidance from leaders; then they will stumble even in daylight. The prophet Hosea was dragged down to the level of the people and stumbled. Perhaps he thought he was safe or immune because of his spiritual standing or reputation, but he is not - he stumbled too.

"You stumble day and night, and the prophets stumble with you. So I will destroy your mother— my people are destroyed from lack of knowledge. Because you have rejected knowledge, I also reject you as my priests; because you have ignored the law of your God, I also will ignore your children."
[9](Hosea 4:5-7)

Vaccinations are wonderful...

When one has a vaccine for a disease, the body reacts as if it were suffering from the full infection.

The white blood cells start producing the antibodies to destroy the virus and to prevent further viral replication[1]. The antibodies can stay in the body and, for some time, individual cells in the immune system 'remember' the antigen (**invading microbe**) and can produce the correct antibody again at short notice - this causes the actual immunity.

Vaccines form a significant part of protecting children and adults from various infectious diseases. After a hundred-year-old battle between the authorities and often unconvinced, sometimes aggressive society, the scepticism has somewhat waned. Over time, we have seen the Industrial Revolution where the slums of especially British cities were breeding grounds for disease; things have improved as civilisation and medical science evolved.

As this evolution plays out and the population becomes more literate, leaflets and pamphlets carry the messages that social media carries today. Placards back then would read like "Vaccination: its fallacies and evils", "Vaccination, a Curse" and the very cryptic "Horrors of Vaccinations"[2]. Today's titles read somewhat differently with similar connotations: "Deadly Conspiracy NHS workers join the anti-vax Facebook group that claims corona virus vaccine is a 'poison' to be 'unleashed' on the world."[3] **(The Sun, 16 Nov 2020)**. "Piers Corbyn, brother of former labour leader Jeremy Corbyn, believes COVID-19 is a 'hoax'" [4] Credit: PA: Press Association (**The Sun, 16 Nov 2020**).

The Polio vaccine is administered orally as a liquid; I remember it like it was yesterday when I got my immunization as a boy. It was an Easter holiday break in a rural village called Lowe River in the parish of Trelawny, Jamaica. During the week leading up to the vaccination day, we as children were terrified. It was customary for us to receive these intravenously in the principal's office. The vaccination day meandered along and 4 pm approached; at 10 minutes to the hour, I hauled myself into the clinic. Nurse Kelly was a neighbour and ran the session, looking after the few people that were present.

"Sit in that chair," she said.

Chapter 1

"Stick out your tongue." she released two drops of liquid onto my waiting tongue. I had my vaccine and could not believe it; my fear of needles had crippled me.

The Measles, Mumps, Rubella (MMR) vaccine used for decades, which protects children against measles, mumps, and rubella, is administered as an injection. It was a welcome initiative in 2007; a breath of fresh air at a time when the Guardian newspaper displayed a bold message that read "MMR is safe. Tell your friends". This article was presented by the scientist, columnist and author Ben Goldacre who disclosed information on the case at the time. He reported the findings by the General Medical Council (GMC) that investigated Andrew Wakefield, disgraced former physician and academic, along with his co-defendants and in January 2010 reported that they failed to meet the high standards expected to be upheld by doctors in research.

In that instance it was reported that Wakefield and his team were guilty of being 'misleading', 'irresponsible' and purely 'dishonest' when they described where children described in a 1998 study into the matter came from. It is alleged that the data came from routine experimental referrals.

A great deal of controversy previously existed over this vaccination and its possible link to autism. Today the original paper has been discredited, and both co-authors have made public statements rejecting its implications. Vaccinations are administered at set intervals during a child's first five years.

The public gives the authorities in charge of health a challenge of massive proportions. A school of thought is that once there is over two-thirds of the community vaccinated, herd immunity develops. Much of this depends on how infectious the disease is as in some cases 50% to 90% of the population requires immunity before infection rates begin to slope downwards[5]. In this case the community (the herd) develops immunity to the disease, making the transfer of the infection from person to person highly unlikely.

This means the society is protected when the next generation has no memory of that microbe's disturbance and threat. People in community swing from the enormous risks of having the disease to much less chance of being protected. Vaccine hesitancy means the virus will meet less resistance as it spread rapidly across communities because of a lack or low immunity[6]. It is not always the case that people are against vaccination, it is more often than not fear and lack of explanation supplied by conversation.

Some of the vaccines claims have allowed society to fall prey to social media and worldwide despot and capitalist leaders. The blame has been laid at the feet of bureaucratic government and also on anti-vaxxer sentiments. Impressionable people all over the world are fed a diet of unleavened lies backed up by a massive dollop of misinformation garnished with disinformation from "Your Auntie Doris' Facebook page..." - @ Mr. Jamesob.

Chapter 1

(Artificially Acquired Passive Immunity)
Active or Passive Vaccination?

Immunity by definition is the body's ability to protect itself from an infectious disease. Being able to fight off a disease or infection is the body defense from inside out. It is either that you're born with it or you acquire it. Innate immunity, also known as natural or genetic immunity, is immunity that an organism is born with. The genes carry the code for fighting particular disease. This genetic immunity protects an organism throughout their entire life. Being born with the immunity means that there are two types of defenses:

First, there is external, otherwise known as the first line of defense, where the work is to protect the organism from exposure to harmful microbes. The skin, stomach acid and tears are examples.

Secondly, there are internal defense (called the second line of defense) that deals with pathogens that get past the first line and enters the body. Included in this are things like inflammations and fevers. Immunity can be adjusted for use in different conditions, also known as acquired immunity. This is the third line of defense and protects an organism from a specific pathogen. This kind breaks down further into two subgroups: active immunity and passive immunity.

Dr. Ramon Arscott, a Bermudan plastic surgeon, explained in very user-friendly language how the vaccine works, having

36

worked on immunity and immunology at the same famous Oxford University in his fascinating YouTube video[1] 'War on Covid'. He likened the immune system to a literal army having a 'General', CD4 helper T-Cell; CD8 killer T-Cells; 'infantry/soldiers' that fights invaders; Antigen Presenting Cells (APC) are the 'detectives' that go around finding the intruders (invaders).

Then there are the regular 'military police 'whose job is to find and 'cuff 'the invaders biologically known as antibodies. When the cells are made in the bone marrow of the human body they are then schooled about the cells making up the body. The lessons are given in a specialized organ known as the Thymus; this organ reduces in size as you get older.

It informs the 'detectives', about the things that make you unique, what makes you the person you are. Once this information is logged, for the rest of your life they survey every cell in your body for any change in the 'blueprint'. When the APCs find' intruders' e.g. a virus they bring them to the 'stations' which are the lymph nodes positioned around the body. 'The General' [CD4 killer T-cells] will decide what will happen to the invading microbe depending on what is known about it. The 'officers' will create specific 'cuffs' in huge numbers having the memory of what the invading microbe is so if it is ever 'seen' in the body again, it is ready to pounce.

Chapter 1

What is active immunity?

This is the kind of immunity in which a pathogen takes place following the exposure to the kind of pathogen (a microbe that causes disease). When the body is exposed to a new [novel] disease agent, B cells, a type of white blood cell, create antibodies that assist in destroying or neutralizing the disease agent. Antibodies are Y-shaped proteins that are able to bind to sites on toxins or other pathogens called antigens. Antibodies are disease-specific, so each antibody protects the body from only one disease agent. An example is, antibodies produced when the body discovers the virus that causes AIDS will not provide any defense against cold or flu viruses.

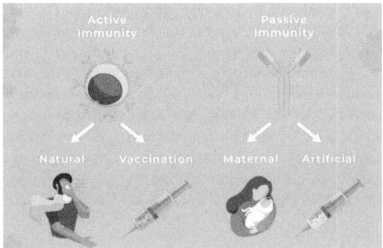

A diagram showing the different types of active and passive immunity[2]

Vaccine Storage/ shortage

Vaccines are stored at low temperatures to prolong their effectiveness and to have them ready in large quantities. Different vaccines require different temperatures; the RNA versions like those produced by Pfizer and Moderna require much colder storage than those made by more established sources[1]. The logistics involved with the rollout of vaccines is the most crucial aspect, and countries with the knowledge of how to do so efficiently and effectively will be ahead of the curve. Societies will be stretched to breaking points because of demand for the COVID -19 vaccines worldwide.

The need for this highly specialised type of storage will render several countries unable to afford certain vaccines because of their remoteness and economic status[2]. Situations like this highlight the disparity between the rich and poor in our society and the need for people to accept shared responsibility. The cold chain can be defined as the transportation of temperature-sensitive products. It can be viewed as a science; it is heavily reliant on assessment and space for the connection between temperature and perishability; a technological feat that for the longest time united global trade.

It relies heavily on several methods to keep the products at the right temperatures; journey times, seasonality, and packaging contribute to the process. All vaccines must be refrigerated and kept from light; freeing them could diminish their efficacy and if they are not kept at the prescribed temperatures the manufacturers will not accept responsibility for any subsequent failure of the product to do what it was designed to do.

All these disciplines are essential to maintain the integrity of the products being moved from the point of manufacture to the end user. A cold chain is not a new phenomenon, but the level of its service will be unprecedented. It has been used to transport food for a long time but the sensitivity and importance of vaccine transportation requires strategic planning. For centuries ice has been used to preserve 'perishable' goods, especially food and fish. The vaccination of millions of people in different parts of the world will require the cold chain to fire at full capacity.

With the approval of several vaccines developed worldwide, it will require the most precise transportation system. Pfizer/ BioNTech are ahead of the rest of the vaccine producers and have managed to create a vaccine with over 90% effectiveness/efficacy during trials across the age range[3]. Some difficulties were storing it at -70 degrees Celsius (-94F) until just before administration and avoiding spillages in transit. Since they are made from RNA (mRNA) molecules held in a liquid nano-particle and can degrade or be otherwise destroyed very easily, the need to store at freezing temperature becomes even more significant.

Think about how we preserve food in our freezers, sometimes for years. The idea is to prevent decomposition; preventing chemical reactions occurring helps to achieve this.

Refrigerated lorries or planes will take the pre-packed boxes of this precious cargo to centralised positions in different countries. Once on-site, they are tested in batches to ensure the quality remains high. On approval the batches are moved to storage vats – big freezers where they are, kept for months, providing the temperature is at -70°C always, and can only be taken out to be defrosted when it is time to use them.

The vaccine was to be transported from Belgium where the manufacturing hub is sited across the British Isles, and we were not to know that this would lead to problems between nations[4] at the time. How this will work is still a mystery as leadership challenges have plagued the UK government. The vaccines from Pfizer are packaged as produced in vials containing five doses or thereabouts. It is interesting to note that they are bathed in a diluted saline solution; the type you would get in a pharmaceutical setting. The vials are then readied for shipping stacked in adapted freezer boxes[5].

Once the vaccine has been checked and approved, another essential aspect begins. Distribution to the masses becomes a difficult task and is not to be frowned at in any way. The way administrators implement the rollout for vaccines remain a most crucial aspect of the fight against COVID-19 and the preparation process remains the first key to its success. Hospital hubs will receive the vaccines worldwide and then manage the administering of it to the people.

Note that it is only mandatory to store the vaccine at the extreme temperature of -70°C for the long term. The hospitals will hold them for a much shorter time and will be able to use regular freezers/fridges. It was thought the vaccine will be suitable for up to a month in these conditions and after delivery, ice is used to preserve it. This would be ideal for up to five days in this condition. Poorer countries would never be able to afford these vaccines because of the logistical burden it carries.

Depending on the area's size, the hospital hubs will distribute the vaccine to the areas that the governments would have prioritised. In the case of the UK, it could be doctors' surgeries and pharmacies. In homes for the aged and other settings, it is possible to transport the vaccine to the patients in a cold transport, temperature 2-8°C. The vaccine then gets defrosted, prepared, and given as an injection into the arm within six hours.

It is only at this point when drug companies can develop a vaccine against the mutated H5N1. So there has been precedence set at several points in the past; vaccine productions in a much shorter time than the typical five to seven years[7]. During pandemics, when all the world's resources for vaccine development concentrate on getting a vaccine that could cause society to return to normality, time is no object. The quickest way to produce such a vaccine is to use biotechnology rather than the chick embryos method; vaccines were produced by inoculating chick embryos with the virus[8].

Valneva based just outside Livingstone in Scotland has reported using the old, tried, tested and proven blueprints for vaccine development to bring through its addition to the 'vaccine fest'. The UK government's vaccine had its hope on

42

being developed by Astra Zeneca in collaboration with Oxford University who used the cold virus from a chimp as the platform for their vaccine. It proved useful in the fight against Ebola in western Africa in the recent past.

Pfizer BioNTech and Moderna - two mRNA vaccine producing companies - joined the vaccination race producing efficient vaccines that are now widely used. Johnson & Johnson, the world-renowned company, brought the first one dose vaccine (Ad 26. COV2.S) to the table and it is confident that all checks will be passed as it prepares its regulatory filings for the global rollout. It baffles me to find that government talk so loosely about the vaccination being the 'cure' for this pandemic, adding to the confusion faced by many in the population. It is down to the lack of education and misinformation on our lawmakers' part and this makes people unsure of what message to accept.

"With 90% efficacy it means that life could return to normal by spring 2021" was a poor messaging on the part of the UK government. The UK having ordered 40 million doses, enough to vaccinate a significant portion of the population, began to lift the mood of many. Boris Johnson has stressed caution, and rightly suggested that people should not rely on the vaccine as a solution, and that we should not slacken our resolve – continue to do the right thing - "Hands, Face, Space and protect the NHS".

One doctor / lawyer who dealt in international medical matters explained that vaccine rollout was an overly complex undertaking. He pointed out to Shelagh Forgathy on her daytime radio show on Leading Britain's Conversation (LBC) that pandemically it was still very precarious. There will be developing countries even now who will not be able to afford the vaccine because of logistics and other considerations. A most concerning drawback is the need for this vaccine to be kept at temperatures as low as -70 °C. Not many countries with experience in pharmaceuticals can deliver vaccines efficiently. India is a typical example, they have much experience in this sector, but poverty and population restraints could prove debilitating even after finding a vaccine.

Fortunately, other vaccines are stored at higher temperatures. Oxford University's offering in partnership with Astra Zeneca can be stored at fridge temperatures, allowing easier distribution and more comfortable access by smaller and lower countries.

The intelligent, educated analysis suggests that if the vaccine is rolled out worldwide and there are pockets of society where there are still epidemic proportions that would lead to the re-entry of the virus into developed nations. Where I am perplexed is the impact this will have on the world at large... Poor countries and their people will continue to be marginalised in commercial and business travel areas. Cost is an issue; the point that is not made enough is that many of these middle- and low-income economies will be marginalised in the vaccination rollout. Industrialised countries with the resources will monopolise the access and procurement of vaccines, making the world a less than secure place.

The World Health Organisation's (WHO) echoes are that no one in the world is safe from the SARS-COV2 virus until the entire world is free from it. The strategy needs to be to ensure that all sections of the globe get access and the Johnson & Johnson vaccine appears to have agreed to deliver up to 100 million doses at the cost of $10 per dose. Comparatively, Pfizer BioNTech is up to around $19.50 per dose and the lower priced AZ vaccine at $4 per dose[9]. Added to that fact, the Oxford Astra Zeneca collaboration was founded on the understanding that poorer countries would get the vaccine at cost price, so no profits made off it until the pandemic is over[10].

Selfishness is a common theme in this corona virus pandemic, collectively as well as individually. Political, wealthy, societies that have travelled around as the main population of countries like Britain are not getting the level of leadership required to get nations out of the current pandemic. I want to bring out the fact that the vaccine is the savior, while in the 'developed world' governments, the ordinary Joe is asked to sit at home unless the need to leave is without compromise. Whether two doses for full protection within reason or one dose is given to as many people as possible for some protection, we need to get it to all the people across the world over age 65 yrs as soon as possible. This age group in the developed world is mostly covered and the hesitancy is mainly from the younger adult population.

Warnings about what will result from the variants in circulation worldwide are coming from experts from all quarters, the most recent being an Indian variant (B.1.617.2 later christened the delta variant identified in the UK[11]. Michael Osterholm, an epidemiologist in America and Director of the Centre for Infectious Disease Research and a member of the new USA president's COVID-19 advisory team, described what can be called a surge in cases in the forecast. On that advice the case for single dose vaccines into as many arms as possible will provide more protection.

Mutations occur all the time in the background but fortunately the variants of the SAR-CoV-2 virus present change slowly. It does not prevent vaccines from helping people but instead will reduce the protection level; all the approved vaccines up to now can provide enough security to the recipient. B117 the code for the Kent variant of the virus that now appears in many countries. Thank goodness, there is no evidence that the mutation in this virus strain affects the ability of the antibodies made by the vaccines to work effectively. Dr Osterholm opines that the virus's ability to 'cause more infections and much more serious illness is there'.

I know many who read these words may not have the technical understanding of the virus's ability to change and the effect of those changes so I will expand briefly on the variants that we know about today. Other variants, for example those observed from South Africa and Brazil, present additional likely fears because they "may evade the immune protection from either natural disease or from the vaccine." (Peter Wade, *Rolling Stone*).

A case made for the latest vaccine in the fight, the one from Jensen - Johnson & Johnson that was trialled widely including areas of the United States and South Africa showed extremely high protection levels. Research shows that no deaths occurred from the South African variant, scientifically that means that at least serious illness from the virus will attenuate (lessen) if not fully protected from it.

A doctor named Anthony spoke to James Obrien about losing his 67-year-old dad to COVID-19, early in the pandemic. Speaking through his tears, Anthony explained how he "prayed". It was his wish to be dead rather than his dad, 'If there's a God out there'. He sounded a broken man, hopeless... I know many people are suffering from pandemic fatigue and serious economic strain, which has led to states and whole countries loosening restrictions on activities like normal schools and indoor dining.

Many believe that opening up society fully will not help the cause; in America for example amidst the chaos of lack of doses and the small scale take up of the vaccine in areas like New York City where the demographic is so varied. Latinos and African Americans make up a large percentage of that population and vaccine resistance is extremely high. Doctors and volunteers address the vaccine misinformation and disinformation; both topics discussed elsewhere in this book.

It was refreshing as a Christian believer to hear a medical doctor utter the following words "I believe there is a God out there who holds the future in his hands" (**Jeremiah 29:11.**)

Social distancing and other precautions must continue because vaccine rollouts take a long time – refrigeration and transport will prove difficult and have far-reaching implications in the world. At this time, the questions are being asked about the way out of the crisis. In some quarters they ask and answer the question of the programme of vaccination and whether it should be made mandatory - (**Swarbrick on Sunday, LBC**)

Restrictions are already in place where they make sense. The Yellow fever vaccine is an example (Samantha Vonvox – Oxford vaccine group.)

Injections vs. pills.

- Polio vaccination (oral)

- MMR is injected; the measles vaccine provides lifelong immunity.

- Influenza injected; vaccine injected and is administered annually even though the virus causing it mutates regularly.

- Tetanus injected.

The vaccine development process used to be extended because of the various checks and balances required. This one has been expedited because of all the resources that are being made available for COVID-19 to be brought under control. There is still the problem of inequality in the world as is seen with the plight of India, Brazil, and other developing economies. The mega-rich countries have monopolised the procurement of vaccines and although India, for example, is the biggest producer in the world and yet they do not have enough for their citizens.

All this happens against the backdrop of the UK boasting the success of their vaccine rollout while many countries in the rest of the world has managed to vaccinate under 5% of their population. India reported that they have exported over 70 million doses of the vaccine during the first four months of 2021; availability of patents for vaccine production would alleviate much of the problem. Western societies like the UK and EU hold the patents and have refused to make them available to developing countries.

Dr. Sarah Jarvis ....Vaccine centre London school of tropical medicine spoke with LBC's Eddie Mair@ 6:30pm Tuesday 20/7/2021 confirming that vaccines are safe; they have been tested in the same way they would have been done pre- Covid-19. This is the biggest vaccination drive in the history of the world. Responsibility…

Research published in the Lancet, a respected source of information on health related matters suggested "We found that the odds of having symptoms for 28 days or more after post - vaccination infection were approximately halved by having two vaccine doses."

Chapter 2

...To mask or not to mask...

Let me start this chapter with an explanation about face masks and carbon dioxide. Normal oxygen saturation levels are in the 95-100% range. This myth must be dispelled in order that the society can rest assured about the efficacy of mask wearing in the war against COVID-19. When a mask and shield is worn for over two hours the pulse oximeter reads 98% and carbon dioxide 33-35% both of which are normal levels.

The scientific explanation is that owing to the size of the molecules of oxygen and carbon dioxide being very tiny the excuse supplied for not wearing the mask does not stand. Droplets, on the other hand, are much bigger are caught in the fabric and as a result protects the wearer from SARS-CoV-2 virus.

Even doctors are hung up on the wearing of masks. It is certainly not comfortable; a surgeon could spend several hours in surgery and wear the mask throughout. They find masks inconvenient; "I'd rather not wear one, I like to see people's faces. I'd rather not bother with it" opines Dr. Greg Schmidt, Intensive care physician. Dr. Schmidt settles the argument by advising that in order to remove the need for face masks in the future we need to wear it now. It's important to wear these face coverings now so we can get our lives back...

Can DIY masks protect you from COVID-19?

The answers are many and varied, depends on whom you are listening to in this situation. The infection is novel, as you are aware, it means it is new. We do not know too much about SARS-CoV-2. It is a new virus; however, the family is not new. Viruses are not newcomers to civilisation; they have been here for a long time; some records suggest up to 30 million years. The world has seen the scattering of a range of viruses in different corners of the globe[1]. Boston College, USA, revealed that a team of scientists was working assiduously on that project as we speak.

The jury is out on how we protect ourselves in this pandemic; wearing a mask is the proverbial football; being kicked around by all. Masks work but they need to be worn and worn properly. One important observation I have is the number of people who wear masks in a way that it does not offer any protection. Wearing a mask under the chin [like a beard] or under the nose is like 'fixing three of the five doors in your submarine…'[2], we must get people to start using these tools right. That would help fight the pandemic in a big way.

It is interesting to note that retroviruses are a large family of viruses that usually cause mild to moderate upper-respiratory tract illnesses, like the common cold. However, three new corona viruses have emerged from animal reservoirs over the past two decades to cause serious and widespread illness and death. Other prevalent viruses include human immune-deficiency virus (HIV -1 and -2) that causes AIDS and Ebola viruses that caused the disease of the same name. These are very topical globally, and many people worldwide have encountered one or more of the many viruses present in nature.

Viruses are very tiny and are parasitic; they need hosts to survive. Unfortunately, the corona viruses have been around long and viruses do not leave fossils behind, and, as such, the information about them and their origin is very sparse. Studies have shown that their genetic sequences accumulate in the DNA genomes of living things, including humans and can leave 'footprints' for discovering the natural history of the symbiotic relationships between them and their hosts.

Corona viruses (so named because of the appearance under the microscope – spiky or crown-like) have surfaced in Asia over the past decade where (severe acute respiratory syndrome) SARS and (Middle East respiratory syndrome) MERS have affected populations adversely. SARS-CoV-2 is the most recent virus to emerge and causes COVID-19, the disease causing the ongoing worldwide pandemic.

Stopping the spread of germs has always been a fundamental rule for keeping populations safe. For COVID-19 and by extension the pandemic to be kept controlled, we must do the following:

- Avoid touching eyes, nose, and mouth.
- Sanitise and disinfect frequently touched objects and surfaces.
- Remember to use soap and water to wash hands for an extended period

- Stay at home when showing signs of illness, except to get medical care.
- *Always wear a mask while in enclosed places and around others, especially where social distancing is challenging to maintain.*

The following facts are (or should be) embedded in our consciousness:

- There are currently no vaccines to prevent COVID -19, but the ones available have proven effective in stopping hospitalization and death.
- To effectively prevent illness is to avoid exposure to the SARS-CoV-2 virus.
- Authorities reckon it is spread mainly from person to person in these ways:
1. Where people are in close contact with one another (within 2 metres, about two arms' lengths)
2. Sputum and other droplets produced when an infected person coughs, sneezes, or talks.
3. The sputum contains droplets that can land in the mouths or noses of people nearby; it is recognised that a point of entry the virus relies on is by inhalation.
4. Studies have revealed that asymptomatic (not showing symptoms) people may spread the disease rapidly.

Wearing a mask is a big issue for some individuals, including world leaders. CDC Director Robert R. Redfield MD opines that the mask is one of the most effective ways of fighting COV19[2, 3]. "I wear a face mask to ensure the COV19 stops with me", he said in a statement to the American people – CDC.

DIY Masks...

The world is awash with people suggesting making your own masks. Social media trends have caught on, and people have been making their masks using t-shirts, scarves, and other materials. When you wear a mask, you essentially want something to protect you, a filter to prevent you from inhaling airborne particles. The cotton is not delicate enough to work as a filter; some say the holes in the fabric are tiny because they do not understand viruses' size.

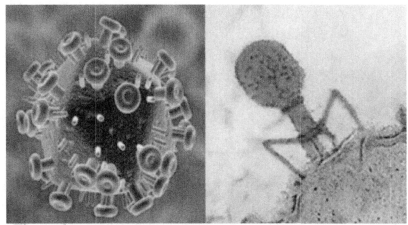

Figure 1: An idea of the virus from an electron micrograph (most vary in diameter from 20 nanometres (nm; 0.0000008 inches) to 250–400 nm)

According to one study from the US national library of medicine, 82% of droplets are expelled from a coughing range of 0.74 -2.12 micrometres[4]. That is about the size of 1/80th of the diameter of a strand of your hair. Suppose we study a chart showing the efficiency of masks made from different materials.

Figure 2: Percentage of particles masks from selected materials can filter out[5]

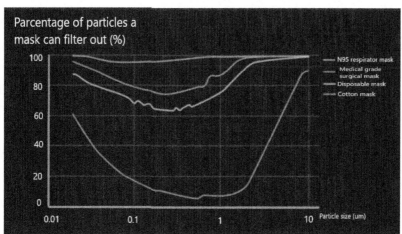

In that case, we find that in a NIOSH research to measure masks results' efficiency. The addition of cotton masks done by researching and finding a chart from the US library of medicine and concluding that they are inefficient and should not be dependable.

The Lancet reported on January 30, 2020, that Roth and colleagues described SARS-CoV-2 in several individuals infected by someone who was said to be asymptomatic and had travelled from China. This report was questioned because the standard case took acetaminophen for jet lag, which can mask symptoms of COVID-19.

Hence, the scientific community has become sceptical about the transmission of infection by asymptomatic individuals. It has since become clear that people are contagious for at least 48 hours before symptoms appear (before symptoms), that some people only have mild (few symptoms) symptoms, and some remain entirely asymptomatic. This showed in these individuals transmitting the virus without knowing they were contagious - the main argument for using face masks as a source control.

Also, there is still controversy over the risks of transmission through volatile SARS-CoV-2. In contrast, these perceived conflicts continue to fuel conflicting advice about the potential role and type of face masks in the COVID-19 pandemic for health care workers and the public. Systematic reviews of face mask use indicate relative reductions in risk (RR) of infection ranging from 6 to 80%, including beta-corona virus disease (for example, COVID-19, SARS, and MERS) [6].

A difference in inclusion and exclusion criteria for the type of studies may lead to this discrepancy in the result. The kind of population covered - such as healthcare workers or the public; maybe the type of face mask used; the outcomes considered, including laboratory-confirmed virus versus symptoms alone, as well as undesirable consequences; and the setting e.g., epidemic versus non-epidemic scenarios. For COVID-19, the evidence of this is presented in an edition of The Lancet [7].

The available evidence is of low or extremely low certainty because it is derived from observational studies with a significant risk of various biases, or indirect evidence from randomised studies of other (non-beta corona) respiratory viruses' methodological limitations [8].

Despite the uncertainty, the range of the potential RR limit must be considered in the local epidemiological context and translated into absolute risk reductions. In Norway, for example, it was estimated that 200,000 people needed to wear face masks to prevent one new infection per week. They assumed a 40% reduction RR with surgical masks[9]. There was a need to avoid this large number due to the low prevalence or risk of infection. From a demographic perspective, one could argue that wearing a face mask would not be worth the public's money and would not outweigh any potential harm.

Deciding to wear a face mask is left to the individual, depending on the values they place on the results[10]. However, in an environment with a high underlying risk, such as healthcare workers caring for a highly prevalent patient with COVID-19, wearing a mask (applying the same relative effect as above) prevents infection in up to one in two.

A strong recommendation that all these individuals wear a face mask may be warranted, despite the uncertainty in the evidence. The stark contrast is the context and the underlying risks, not the difference in the relative effect that face masks provide. Time will tell, but it is not yet clear where the exact threshold is for the real risks that justify the use of face masks in society. The description of the thing as a "face-nappy" has caused many people to avoid following the rules (or their mandate) foolishly.

Given the paucity of evidence for serious adverse effects from invasive interventions, wearing a face mask may be acceptable in many situations, although more evidence is needed. That evidence is continuing to unfold as the pandemic rages on; many countries have entered second and third lockdowns because of the high levels of infection.

Where does this leave us even at the height of this pandemic? Acknowledging the current uncertainty about the quality of the evidence and understanding the difference between relative and absolute reductions in risk is central to sorting out the many questions and confusion about face masks. They can make recommendations and policymakers make decisions about the type of face mask, which is influenced by underlying risk, cost, fairness, acceptability, and feasibility. However, they must be transparent about the context and criteria that they consider in their recommendations.

Public health measures to implement face mask use will be more important in increasing the baseline risk of transmission. There is evidence of beneficial effects in studies of medical masks, and such products may also exist for perfectly designed cloth masks. However, direct evidence is currently limited to observational and droplet studies[11].

No single intervention gives invulnerability to SARS – CoV-2. From a public health standpoint, it is essential to stress the importance of other risk mitigation strategies to reduce the number. Others include proximity, duration of personal contacts, respiratory, hand hygiene measures, and engineering measures in built environments. Using a face mask should not be a substitute for these risk mitigation strategies, but it may be beneficial. For example, it might not be easy to maintain physical distancing in high baseline risk settings, such as work and school environments.

Double masking evolved into 'a thing', it is when one mask is worn on top of the other helping to improve the fit and efficiency of filtration of the mask. The CDC in America produced a study that concluded that double masking effectively prevented the sprays generated from breathing, speaking, and coughing[12]. It is important to note also that there needs to be a specific combination of masks, a cloth mask over a surgical mask was the advice. Other combinations proved not as effective, if at all. It is useful to test out your double mask in your home before going out, this ensures it fits well and your breathing and sight are not hampered[13]

Future steps should include conducting high-quality studies, including the use of standardised cloth masks for some people, especially in western countries for both, the estimates of effects and contextual factors in tandem with ongoing evidence synthesis. Nations and nationals must work together to promote efforts to combat polemicism and division for rapid scientific advancement to address the current global crisis. Some researchers argue that people are unlikely to wear masks properly or consistently, and may ignore wider infection control measures like hand washing. Others say the public should not wear them since healthcare workers need them more[14].

In this regard, governments Norway and Canadian have funded initiatives that map the evidence and will provide a trusted catalogue[15], including for mask-use whilst pondering and will provide information to allow navigation in different conditions.

Such a catalogue will be strengthened by controlled trials of facemask use (e.g. NCT04337541)[16].

Benefits of DIY masks include the availability of common materials, the lower risks posed by people without symptoms shedding viral loads through speaking, coughing, and sneezing. Where it is difficult to maintain social distancing DIY masks offer some protection. These are not without drawbacks, that include the feeling of a false sense of safety, forgetting that protection from these face coverings is limited. There are studies that claim they are 50% less helpful in preventing infections than surgical N95 respirators. My conclusion is that these measures do not work in isolation and consistent proper hygiene practices and reduced physical contact combine to offer the best protection possible.

Nevertheless, the results of the available experiments should not lead to a fruitless return to the ongoing debate between the risk of adherence bias, contamination, and applicability of the results. Indeed, these studies should prevent reliance on environmental data that cannot determine causation. They should provide the required quantitative estimates that highly controlled laboratory studies cannot provide despite their value in understanding transmission.

Anti–Maskers

There are many good reasons why we would opt out of wearing masks if we could get away with it. Masks pick up dust, trigger allergies, cause itchiness and possibly 'make' mask induced acne. When you wear a mask for long enough, the strings cause the backs of your ears become tender and raw. Also, without an extender that keeps your mask secure, having a loose mask is tantamount to wearing no mask at all. Wait, if this is, we were miserable last summer when it was not mandatory in many countries when we return to that season next year and must wear the mask, wow!

I spoke to a young woman recently on her way from the UK to Jamaica for four weeks. I wished her well and said she should make sure she had her mask, and her response was typical. She said she packed more masks than clothes, masks in all styles and patterns. Different colours, sizes, styles, masks have come very far!

All the inconveniencies of mask-wearing could be nothing compared to what might be the case if you found out it could damage your lungs in any way. The question still begs; social media and conspirators have spread the gospel of the anti-maskers as the pandemic raged. Names like '*face nappies*' and '*muzzles*' conveyed the message of dissatisfaction.

The claims that health may be compromised circulated in spring 2020 only months after the world stood up to take notice of COVID-19 pandemic; this was around the time different organisations recommended using face coverings to prevent the spread. Asian societies have experienced respiratory diseases like SARS and MERS and we hold them up as examples[1].

South Korea, Taiwan and Singapore were singled out for special praise, and the low rate of spread vindicated the claim. However, it is still a school of thought that if one wears a mask for long periods, one runs the risk of hypercapnia or 'carbon dioxide poisoning' (excess of carbon dioxide in the blood), something I argued elsewhere in this book[2]. I know from research, and real-life examples, of surgeons during lengthy procedures wear their surgical masks for extended periods with no ill effects on their carbon dioxide retention.

If that were possible, then it would be devastating the effects of a surgeon with a reformed mental state whilst performing the long operation on the brain of an 'anti-masker'. There is also no evidence of mask-wearing, causing hypoxemia, which affects the arteries[3]. These arteries are the blood vessels that carry blood to cells (*Dr Daniel Diaz; National Autonomous University of Mexico medical school*). Dr Diaz's opinion is that the lack of information may come from the feeling people are afraid of their airflow blocked, which may be due to the masks' material. He reassures us that that feeling is mostly because the general population not used to wear the covering, but prolonged use would solve that problem.

Society needs to understand that there is more to gain than lose from wearing masks. Organisations such as the CDC in USA and SAGE in the UK, PAHO/WHO (Pan American Health Organization/ World Health Organization) in the Caribbean are leading the efforts in the region are leading in the advising the masses on the appropriate use of face coverings in the fight against COVID-19. With that said, there are categories of people who will not benefit from mask-wearing.

A typical group would be children under two years old and those suffering from respiratory/ breathing problems. It is difficult, but there are schools of thought in which some medical professionals are of the view that even people with conditions that are usually protected, e.g. sufferers from asthma or COPD (chronic obtrusive pulmonary disorder) should wear a face-covering where possible (Professor *Neil Schachter – Mount Sinai hospital*). The professor, earlier this year, pointed out that we must protect those with compromised airways.

My next-door neighbour had orders to quarantine for several weeks during the first wave of the pandemic because he suffers from one such condition and is over 70 years old. He has now sadly passed on, though not with COVID-19 as he had both of his jabs prior to this death.

The fly in the ointment is around the fact that information is in short supply, and the little around is tainted by the users of social media platforms and the ease with which the 'share-aholics' just hit send. Many ignorant people and other with the fear agenda have caused confusion in many communities.

Some 'Youtubers' are enjoying a bumper season peddling misinformation[4],(https://www.youtube.com/watch?v=ciYFgVp ya5k) making a killing out of the misery attributed to a virus who thought that humanity had chosen death (no pun intended here). Big corporations that form the monster's backbone I describe; government advice is mish-mashed at best and tyrannical at worst. The crisis's treatment by the "most powerful country in the world" bears testament to this. The truth is, in places like the United States, the Washington Times reported "...it would be far better to have the feds led by President Donald Trump dictating corona virus mitigation than these governors[5].

However, the hard place was; calling for Trump to step in and stop the madness means calling for an end to a constitutional foundation that had already been far too violated by far-leftists trying to stretch their powers, far too many times".

Health care professionals across all borders and sectors are wearers of face-covering; they need PPE, and we go up in arms if they report a lack. These 'soldiers' are called upon to wear this gear for hours on end, shift after shift, after a change in the quest to keep us safe. It escapes me then that society is still opposing the wearing of the protection we can afford. It is not all about protecting ourselves, but our families, friends and neighbours from a disease that knows no boundaries.

To round up this chapter, as we prepare for the 'new normal', wearing face coverings may represent our unified stance in the war against the common threat and reinforce the importance of other measures of social distancing. The recommendations for wearing a face covering are beneficial in the reduction in spread of novel corona virus and COVID-19. The Centre for Disease Control recommends that the covering must protect the nose and mouth when out in the population. Global geography and the current pandemic situation validate the undesirable costs, largely cosmetic; of wearing a face covering may or may not be enough to outweigh the desirable consequences.

Countries ought to put together a massive public education campaign to eliminate the virus. We only need to look to the poliomyelitis disease that was rampant in my grandparents' prime. They saw their classmates and friends in the community die from this crippling disease.

Vaccination was the saviour then, and now it probably is again. In the meantime, we ought to look to the Spanish flu pandemic in 1918 seems a long time ago over 100 years. We could take from the cruel episode from the history books' pages that masks were worn as a barrier even then. These considerations should influence policymakers' recommendations and responsibility by all needs to be the platform from which to build. All parties need to have ownership of the solution led to the involvement of all the relevant stakeholders.

The demographics in cities with high population density in countries like USA, India, Brazil, and South Africa dictate that mask usage will slow and squash the virus. If we look at it by regions like The Americas, Europe, South East Asia, Eastern Mediterranean, Africa then the Western Pacific reveal the confirmed cases numbers in order at the time of writing this — the use of masks will probably outweigh any potential downsides. Viruses mutate or change all the time, usually because of evolution.

Chapter 2

The virus needs to change to survive under pressure from lockdowns, hand-sanitising, social distancing, and vaccinations. It is the case that the SARS-CoV-2 virus that causes COVID-19. Trails over the months have shown that if the entire population wants to contribute to reducing transmission, then a few months of everyone wearing face coverings could contribute to suppression and eventual victory over the virus, even if at the cost of some inconveniences. The temporary loss of some freedoms (transactional fees) might be lower than not responsibly reopening colleges, taking pressure off health care, businesses and schools once standard risk falls to levels that could be considered acceptable.

We need to be careful to understand that no matter how much effort we put in as factions, we are stronger together and whereas there is not a full shield against infection, there is a mixture of measures that will always be required to fight this and any other pandemic.

Studies have shown that masks have been proving effective for many years suggest they helped people with seasonal flu reduce the spread of the virus when they exhaled droplets. Some research evidence points to masks reducing the spread of virus loads into the air. The analysis of another set of study data conducted on Japanese school aged children concluded that vaccination and the wearing of a mask curtailed the chance of developing seasonal flu. It was also found the confirmed that flu rates were minimised when paired with good hygiene.

China: Victim or villain?

It is believed that China covered up the fact that the outbreak of COVID-19 started in Wuhan months before it was announced by the World Health Organisation (WHO). Around February 2020 saw the spread across the world. In America, SARS -CoV 2,which causes COVID-19, had officially claimed over thirteen hundred lives and over sixty thousand infections were recorded. (Bruce Y. Lee, "Cases of COVID-19 jumped due to change in counting method, Forbes, February 13, 2020…")[1].

Make a note here that the real numbers were significantly higher because as you might imagine many died at home and no report made to the agencies, the figures increased exponentially for an extended period with the virus being brought under control.

Another critical factor was the notion that emerged from the reports around the world that deaths that were reported as COVID-19 deaths were untested and potentially were unrelated. Countries including the USA and UK banned travel from China; the USA did so on January 31, 2020. The news outlets there that were saying that the outbreak was not alarming at first were beginning to provide exposés that China might be covering up. The disunited kingdom as it was turning out to be in the unfolding pandemic was less proactive in part; fractious one might say. By February 5, 2020 news broke of details of a second evacuation flight from mainland China; Wuhan specifically was scheduled.

Chapter 2

Caution was given from the (FCO) Foreign and Commonwealth Office to Britons to avoid travel to areas like Hubei Province but only essential travel to the mainland; Macao and Hong Kong were exempted[2]. It was further advised that anyone in China that was able to leave should. At that point in the proceedings, it was hinted that the elderly and people suffering from pre-existing conditions were at a greater risk.

At around this time, conspiracy theories started to unfold, and social media became awash with fantastic stories. Sources close to an evangelical firebrand in the states had given him the scoops on the Chinese connection. One reported that the contact had received information from friends in China that at face value sounded like a major conspiracy theory.

Simply put he believed he had concrete proof that the virus did not come from the wet market where bats and snakes were sold for human consumption, as was reported at the time in 2019, but instead from Wuhan, which was a hub for virology. Hundreds of viruses were collected with the idea of finding vaccines or learning enough to prevent another SARS, MERS, bird flu or swine flu outbreak.

The world was actively trying to understand how these diseases could be handled before they showed up. It was interesting to us who were following the story that there was a rumour the military wanted to use it for biological warfare... or may it just be a conspiracy theory (something suggested as a reasonable explanation for facts, a condition, or an event)[3]. Something went catastrophically wrong, and the virus escaped. Seriously weak security mechanism in the Chinese bio lab was then alerted about this time. People were purporting to have names of scientists who "leaked" the news to the world. The word at the time and still now was that the Chinese Communist Party was harbouring a cover-up.

Evangelical journalists, especially on the Charisma news channel in the USA lay claim to be the channel that "informs believers with news for a Spirit-filled perspective... since 1975". The source I refer to claimed that they wanted to report this theory on the channel because of its claims of reporting worldwide spiritual happenings the secular news media refuse to cover. This hot item was not written then because there was no way of verifying or proving its truthfulness according to the source.

Steve Strang [4] wrote that he received an incredibly detailed and exciting text from a friend he called Frank at the time that he believed was authentic, but when he inquired of his friend about the source, it came from another friend called Jay and a number for Jay was provided. Jay confirmed what Frank told Steve during a telephone conversation. But there was still no way of checking the information, apart from travelling to Wuhan or having someone there that spoke the language and was aware of the culture. Although even if this was remotely possible, there was the small matter of the governmental, the Chinese Communist Party ... trying to cover up the truth?

Later sources out of China reported that the SARS-COV -2 virus which I refer to here as the scourge was completely rogue and there was nothing anyone this side of the globe could do about it. Can anyone see the maze that is created here? This is without a doubt what the internet and the social media offerings have done to provide misinformation and disinformation for some time now. My call to the society to take responsibility is borne of this kind of evidence.

Rumours about how the outbreak started became turbocharged by mid-February 2020. We are led to believe that in the beginning the World Health Organisation (WHO) and China put out on the record that the SARS-CoV-2 virus was controllable and could not be passed on through human contact; boy were we misled! By this time, many inhabitants in Wuhan were dead or dying of this respiratory illness.

However, the dictatorship there, as far as we know, does not have issues to do not quarantine rules; the populace was left to get on with it. We saw that it was not until January 23, 2020, that the central government of China imposed the first lockdown in Hubei province. It was referred to as the Wuhan quarantine by the rest of the world as by now we were saturated by the idea that that was where everything came from. Even then the president wanted to ensure that the impression the society at large had was that there was calm.

The Chinese New Year was imminent, and people were not even mandated to wear masks during the celebrations. By early February, according to this source, the scourge was completely rampant, and there was no control, but no responsibility was being taken by those in authority. Many things we were not a party to at the time or that we thought were outlandish are now common knowledge. Christianity in China has been in the news of late; it is even believed that it is the place in the world where the movement is growing at the fastest rate. I am led to believe that at the time in February it was the poorer, marginalised faction of the very densely populated (eleven million people) part of the country that was most affected... Poverty?

The neighboring city of Beijing previously Peking only 720 miles away was not affected in the same way as Wuhan. The conspiracy theorists offer that it was down to the fact that it is the home of six UNESCO heritage sites, the second largest city, and the cultural hub of China. Shanghai is the biggest city in the world and the financial centre of the world, making it a place worth protecting. Both these Chinese cities are nearer to Wuhan China than Rome or Barcelona, yet the outbreak affected the western cities in a much more devastating manner.

Much of what was coming out to the world at the time out the attack was contrary; the leading news media and social media had vastly different accounts of the goings-on. There was a report that the following was unfolding, and it made my source, without any way of confirming the date, take notice. It alleged that a secret lab knew before that the SAR-CoV-2 virus was transmissible by human contact a point I have written about in another part of this book.

Corruption was mooted as a reason for the cover-up, and this was unmasked in January that supposedly involved the government and the Red Cross in Wuhan, which had collected large sums of money but distributed next to nothing. This was rumoured to be over five hundred million Yuan (pronounced

Chapter 2

U- en and the sign for it is ¥) Chinese currency, none of this money reached the people. This led to Red Cross officials losing their positions according to the source.

This was on the heels of the Red Cross losing credibility when officials reported having tarnished its reputation in China when the earthquake recovery was undertaken in 2013. BBC News reported that they fought to "win back trust" after the shambles that occurred in 2008; another quake had hit the mainland and US $12.4 billion in goods and services were donated to the victims.

The news agency reported that the money for the rebuilding efforts was mismanaged by the officials of the Red Cross in China who needlessly purchased expensive tents and vehicles. Research undertaken by the Tsinghua University revealed that 80% of charitable donations after the 2008 Sichuan earthquake were funneled into Chinese government coffers as "extra revenue".[5] In April 2011, according to the source, the Red Cross threw elaborate banquets costing 10,000 Yuan ($ 1,600, £10590) at the time, attended by officials employed by a charitable organisation.

China is still seen as dealing questionably in many of its initiatives, and that is obvious even now. There is the ongoing insistence in Taiwan becoming part of the Chinese republic is one example. President Xi Jinping, in his first speech on January 2, 2019, expressed to Taiwan the fact it had no choice but to become part of the republic. His words were "China must be, will be reunified".[6] The commemorating of compatriots in Taiwan gave Xi a platform from which to trumpet the need and determination for the mainland to be 'One China'.

His statement extended to imply that force is an option that has not been ruled out. The leader of the Chinese continued, "We do not promise to renounce the use of force and reserve the option to take all necessary means". He appeared to be on a war footing and a report from the New York Times said he received moving applause for his combative stance.

At the time, when he first took office the belligerence in his speech in Taiwan gave the impression of the mood in Beijing, China's capital. The attitude in China from then on has been one of unprovoked combat talk. I have mentioned the mustering of biological artillery elsewhere in this book. It was around this time that the USA Navy was to be attacked on the command of a senior officer, Rear Adm. Luo Yuan of the People's Liberation. "The United States is most afraid of death," he said in December 2018 to an audience in the southern Chinese city of Shenzhen. Yuan was very deliberate in his ambition, using provocative language and quoting the number of casualties the USA could have if they were to be hit by the new "aircraft carrier killers" of China.

The ruling Communist Party officials talked of the outbreak starting in Wuhan's wet market spreading via seafood and other exotic food. However, it was immediately disinfected and scrubbed free of any evidence. That was a critical error in procedure but a classic party trick of the Communist Party – please pardon the pun.

Chapter 2

It turned out that the first person to be infected with SARS-CoV-2 had not even been to the market. It was also intimated that a third of the early 41 infections had never been to the fateful wet market. Most of those who had gone never consumed snakes or bats during that period... it appear the excuse of the source of the scourge was fast evaporating. The lab leak theory was gaining traction, there was definitely a link between the Anthony Fauci led coalition "crushed the Donald Trump's theory on the origins of the corona virus" stated CNN.

Peter Dazak working with the EcoHealth alliance also rubbished the claims by Trump's regime. He explained away the theory and promoted the animal-human line while at the same time described the then USA president's allegation as 'pure baloney' at the time. At the same time, scientists developed suspicions about the lab's security, a theory the Donald Trump administration continued to push in the weeks of late march, early April 2020.

Scientist is Dr Li Wenlaing, a Chinese ophthalmologist who was among the first to bring this to the attention of the world through his Weibo posts. [6] It was, in fact, the top chemical and biological lab; believe it or not, the epicentre of the "Wuhan virus" according to Donald Trump is still a working virology lab. The project was a joint venture between France and China in response partially to the SARS outbreak in 2003 to be used for charitable purposes and not as a 'war room'.

As the project unfolded and reached its final knockings, the Chinese government stepped in and took France out of the equation by preventing further participation. Later it was discovered that the Chinese had duplicated the original lab under contract to have three labs like the P4 lab equipped to handle highly contagious pathogens. The Wuhan lab was the hub for Virus Culture Collection and held more than 1,500 strains according to their website. It is a maximum security because of the original P4 lab contract; these viruses were very highly contagious.

It was highly probably that a leak could have occurred because we knew that SARS escaped from labs before; there is record of around six times including from labs in Singapore and Taiwan but astonishing four times from Chinese labs. UK labs were recorded to have lost smallpox viruses at one point killing eighty people; so lab leaks were not novel (pun intended).

Lab leaks have been with us down the years, history records foot and mouth disease striking the Surrey farms in 2007. Professor Nigel Ferguson a renowned modeler of disease spread based at Imperial College London said "We are not completely sure yet, but tit look a laboratory release". I will outline a list of documented leaks taken from a former USA today journalist Alison Young for emphasis:

"Hundreds of bioterror lab mishaps cloaked in secrecy" (17/08/2014)

"Worker at Tulane possibly exposed to bioterror bacteria" (11/03/2015)

"CDC failed to disclose lab incidents with bioterror pathogens to Congress" (23/06/2016)

Chapter 2

"GAO finds gaps in oversight of bioterror germs in U.S"

It is true the those put in to police these programmes have no clue how regularly labs working with many of the world's most lethal microorganisms are failing to fully kill vials of specimens and make them safe before sending them to other research colleagues. Some of these researchers lack the correct equipment to protect them against infection; this came out of a report September 21st 2016, produced by GAO (Government Accountability office. There is form with these agencies and multinational collaboration is a regular thing between them.

In 2015, an international group researcher published a paper on whether a corona virus from bats could infect if manipulated. They worked on a hybrid virus where they combined the SARS virus of two years earlier grown in mice and imitated human disease with the bat virus; this gave oxygen to the theory of viral manipulation in Wuhan. My motive for mentioning these points is not because they were ever verified, but because I know it will interest the reader and provide some background.

In January 2020, guess who was among the first to cast suspicion on the SARS-CoV-2? It was a retired military officer who happened to be Jewish and who worked in the P4 lab for four years, and inside by my definition. Mid-January came around and another group of scientists, this time of Indian descent, told the world that the SARS-CoV-2 is a combination of different viruses, a cocktail. The bat virus referred to as SARS here is the daddy. It has been modified/engineered genetically and mixed with Ebola and HIV... cocktail indeed.

Evidence from those working on the novel corona virus about which I have written elsewhere in this book.

The world was taking notice; Canada, for example, had initiated an investigation in this regard. A Chinese female scientist has been arrested in that country. This individual had covertly returned corona virus from Canada, and it is alleged that she took the virus to the P4 facility in Wuhan China without notifying the authorities in Canada. The travelling public was showing a pattern; Chinese students, businesspeople and immigrants were under the microscope. One case was of a student in Boston who secretly brought the virus to Wuhan and when questioned about who funded her travel did not disclose it.

Research from the head of the corona virus research group of the P4 lab, S Z said that experimental results revealed that there is a significant protein on the human lung cells that serves as a lock mechanism however on the viruses it can serve as a critical mechanism that unlocks the lung cell and allows the virus to enter. I have written about the fallout of this in this book. The researcher indicates that it is a simple process that only replaces four amino acid molecules for this to happen.

Scientists were dying as well; in Canada, there was also the mention of a Kenyan whom I will call Dr Cee, who was reported to have been killed by the virus in Kenya on February 7, 2020. By this time, the world woke up to the fact that the SARS-CoV-2 scourge was global.

Chapter 2

Then President Trump had taken the step and closed the borders, and he got plaudits from sections of the world apart from his power base in the USA in this election year. The evangelicals were firmly in his corner, cheering every decision, good or wrong. On commentator stated that 'Trump doesn't always display the fruits of the Spirit, but the scripture taught us to judge a person by their actions'. Some claimed to see the Lord's hand in the proceedings, a sentiment echoed by the then American president. He also had a *lot* to say about where the virus originated and what the Chinese government was planning.

The musings were coming out of China, particularly from the connection Steve Strang speaks about in his book "God, Trump and COVID". Jay, Steve's contact, said.

"Unfortunately, the Communist Party never spoke the truth. Due to many patients in Wuhan's early days, only a fraction of patients could see doctors. All the hospitals were lacking equipment and other medical resources. Patients were advised to go home to quarantine themselves. So many families all died at home. Per other experts 'estimates, the real number of deaths could be one hundred times more than what was published on government websites. [That is because] official numbers were only from hospitals. Why did this happen to China? This disaster is permitted by God to allow the government to make two major mistakes:

- Ethical issues. Under government blessing, the lead researcher took the lead to research the 'coronavirus'. She had a joint venture with a US private firm. The goal was to research a mechanism to prevent the spread of the corona virus effectively. It was to save lives. But she found a cheap, quick way to turn the corona virus into a much more virulent and more comfortable to spread and attack human beings, version. That private firm considered it very unethical and abruptly stopped the funding and withdrew from the joint venture.

Too much blood on the Chinese 'mainland' was rhetoric. Through seventy years of the reign of the Communist Party, experts estimated that more than 95 million people died in various revolutions or movements in China. That is the biggest battleground between freedom and dictatorship. China has too much "hatred". Jesus' love is something new. It has never been in people's minds. It is unthinkable to many non-Christian Chinese. God has His Time. He has stirred China for His glory. We estimate there are almost 900 million Chinese Christians.

They are hidden currently, operating 'underground'. God is working. Dr Li Wenliang was a seeker of the Christian faith" a house church in Wuhan [Author note: Li Wenliang was the whistle-blower who raised concerns about COVID-19 in December 2019, the disease he died from.] We can see leaked YouTube videos of some Christians in Wuhan passing out flyers and free masks and preaching the gospel on the streets. People and government officials accepted in tears. The government doesn't care, or doesn't know how to care, but the children of God do…

I found that extreme; it is difficult for me to unpack what Jay told Steve Strang [in Trump, God and COVID] those lines entirely. One thing is for sure "Jesus" is in China. My research on the matter and my Christian faith suggest that China's mood is one of acceptance of the growing Christian influence in society. I have mentioned that the faster-growing religion in the world is Islam, followed by Christianity, and much of the Christian growth is in the Republic of China. Research from Pew Research in 2017 suggests the following:

- The Christian population in the world is expected to be 2-9 billion in the next 23 years.

- Christians will remain the world's largest in 2060 reaching numbers of between 3.05 billion or 31.8% [7.]

Interestingly, fertility rates and the current youth population size show the changing profile of the religious demographics for the next forty years. My projections are that Christians will keep the title of the largest religious group; Islam will grow faster than any other major group.[8.] It is a thought that by 2050 the number of Muslims will be the same as Christians around the globe. Atheists, agnostics, and others without affiliations to religious groups '[nones'] will increase in the more prominent western societies like the USA, France and others will make the dwindling portion of the world's population.

Returning to the Chinese influence, as the pandemic meandered on, the lens was trained on the USA yet again, the conspiracy theory in the foreground still. United States senator Tom Cotton began demanding an inquiry as reported in an article in the Wall Street Journal. His opinion was "Beijing has claimed that the virus originated in a Wuhan 'wet market', where wild animals were sold. But evidence to counter this theory emerged in January [9]. Chinese researchers reported in *The Lancet* on January 24, 2020, that the first known cases contact never been in contact with the market, a finding accepted by Chinese state media. There's no evidence pointing to the market selling bats or pangolins, the animals from which the virus is thought to have jumped to humans, and the bat species that carries it isn't found within one hundred miles of Wuhan"[10].

The *National Review* reported the following, "Wuhan has two labs where we know bats and humans interacted. One in the Institute of Virology, eight miles from the wet market, the other is the Wuhan Centre for Disease Control and Prevention, barely three hundred yards from the market"[11]. Senator Tom Cotton was in no doubt China was complicit in the spread of the virus around the world because they knew about the person-to-person transmission since the end of 2019.

They allowed the continuation of international travel. The Senator further reviewed and opined on national television that "this evidence is anecdotal, to be sure, but it all points towards the Wuhan labs," as he concluded in his *Journal* op-ed[12]. "Thanks to the Chinese cover-up, we may never have direct, conclusive evidence; intelligence rarely works in this way–but Americans justifiably can use common sense to follow the inherent logic of events to their likely conclusion." [13.]

Chapter 2

SARS (Severe Acute Respiratory Syndrome) having broken out in the Far East originated in China in 2002 and 2003, and it appeared as though SARS-CoV-2 was showing the same signs in 2019. The SARS epidemic took 774 lives worldwide[14] of which 229 were in Hong Kong[14], causing a mammoth economic slowdown with the stock market, and property markets taking a battering. There were two self-limiting outbreaks around 2002 and 2004 that resulted in a highly transmissible life -threatening type of pneumonia.

After originating in China and then spreading to Hong Kong, the massive spread of SARS was subject to a cover up. It was the same communist regime in power at the time. The question is, could the COVID-19 outbreak another case where China through its dictatorial rule preventing the truth from coming out? History repeated...

The entire world of academics and scientists has fronted up to this COVID-19 pandemic to the extent to which vaccines are developed at mind-boggling rates. However, in the People's Republic of China, many are preoccupied with demonstrating freedom of expression, especially freedom of speech. The truth of what happened in Wuhan was kept under a lid because China has a very stringent system of scoring its citizens, giving societal behaviour points.

In the recent past, it has been implemented much more, and people feared getting low scores as it would adversely affect their social status. They would be marginalised and their families with them. However, there has been a voice of defiance coming in the distance, and some are now gathering the courage to speak out against the oppression handed down by the Chinese dictatorship.

The people could not find jobs, but reports are a revival in the church, probably because of the fear of death from the disease. Christianity arose in a society where the masses were of Chinese descent. The folk religion was practiced, which included Confucian, Taoist doctrines, and Buddhism.

In extreme cases, the movement in China, where Christians are taking to the streets in the face of individual punishment and death, is gaining traction. Some of the officials in the area where the virus is supposed to have started to spread were relieved of their positions. This and other signs suggest the embers of hope are not lying dormant in the coal pot anymore, but they are flickering to light. It is not absolute. We may have a bright future, and an awakening of biblical proportions, but in the meantime, we can pray that the pandemic with catalysing lasting freedom allows for the spreading of the gospel of Christ.

Seeds of the truth are bursting out of the ground in Wuhan, Zhejiang, Fujian, Henan, Shanghai, Hong Kong, North and South Korea where the Rev. John Kim that defected from North to South and is now a pastor in Seoul. At certain points along the North Korean border, several missionaries are reported to have placed them and their converts from North Korea in grave danger. A report further stated that in the recent past, about ten of those in the Christian mission's forefront had died mysteriously; this is the account from Rev. Kim Kyou Ho, a South Korean leader.

Chapter 2

The group is based along the North Korean border called CPN (Chosen People Network) [15]. The name of this organisation fascinates me because these people are pushing on with the message of salvation during the battle. This group is said to run a memorial hall in South Korea for victims who were supposedly killed by North Koreans.

Hundreds of other missionaries have been imprisoned or expelled by China, a country that bans foreigners from proselytizing (evangelising) [16].

Just like it was with SARS and more recently MERS all those years; the word came to us in the west that people were being healed of the SARS-COV -2 virus. Christian believers were getting breakthroughs from praying and worshipping God. The Holy Spirit was doing the work, as the people showed faith in God.

What can we do?

The truth about immunity and immunisation

The need for structured communication has never been greater, lacking from the start of the pandemic, and it has only gotten worse. Governments and other societal leaders have avoided the responsibility of giving the people the clear, concise facts required in emergencies. Church ministers and those in political office are in some cases, guilty of misleading propaganda. The psychology of the pandemic has not been fully understood and nations have been fed with fake news. Knowledge of how a vaccine works is not complicated; they

84

have managed to reduce and in cases eliminate some of the world's deadliest diseases over the last several decades. Polio, measles, and smallpox are just a few that comes readily to mind.

The world faces some conditions right now that are beyond the reach of medical vaccines as we know them, they behave like viruses causing and adding to diseases. Fake news has been weaponised, seasoned with misinformation and spread like a virus across all social and other media networks. Unfortunately, fake stories are so persistent "if you try to debunk it, misinformation sticks with people," says Professor Sander Van der Linden [a psychologist who leads the Social Decision-making Laboratory, University of Cambridge] "Once it becomes integrated into the long-term memory, it is difficult to correct it" he continued.

The immune system is what helps us keep safe. Corona viruses have been around forever; they have been causing diseases like seasonal influenza [flu] and the common cold. The immune system is a defense system releasing cytokines [number of substances, secreted by certain cells of the immune system and affect other cells]. It is also a fact that there can be an adverse effect; there can be super priming or what is known in the virology community called cytokines storm. Flu and other respiratory diseases are caused by corona viruses when the body is attacked the go into attack mode, and lymph nodes swell up while the body fights. The immune system sends fighters to the site and overwhelms the area, e.g., lungs when foreign antigens enter.

Chapter 2

Increase in immune stress in the body caused by stress and poor nutrition–watch your food. Home immunity test questions:

- ✓ How is your energy level today?

- ✓ How clear is your thinking today (7 days fogginess in a day)?

- ✓ How is my digestive tract? – We ought to make sure our diet caters for the colon.

- ✓ My joints – discomfort for more than three days

- ✓ Combine score of over 20 checks.

- ✓ Blood oxygen level needs to be checked – silent hypoxia – pulse oximeter 94%

- ✓ A small bit of alcohol may be suitable for your immune system.

- ✓ Binge drinking is defined as 5-6 glasses of wine.

- ✓ Experiment – half a bottle of Prosecco

Blood sample before and after a binge – Dr Ronx Ikharia (BBC) The drink substantially decreases the number of lymphocytes after the binge drinking between 30-50%. Generally, you are more prone to infections. However, it is true that if we take regular breaks from drinking alcohol, it gives the immune cells time to bounce back.

Neutrophil (first responders) **Lymphocyte** (memory cells) Ratio 3:1 three neuropils to one lymphocyte (NLR) test. Between 1 and 3 is the best result. Gut health is important [our microbiome is essential] 38 trillion of these all over our bodies.

For a tribe of hunter-gathers in Tanzania (Hadza), their food is remarkably diverse, giving a wide range of gut bacteria. A study published in 2017 suggests that they eat mainly from the forest. Fibre is essential, around 30 grams a day. Butyrate is produced when we eat food rich in fibre. This protects macrophages [a type of white blood cell that surrounds and kills microorganisms] in our gut.

Stress has a bad reputation, and the jury is still out as it may have some excellent benefits. Fight or flight is a good example; it is a survival mechanism that is designed to protect the individual. If one fears spiders for instance, and suddenly encounters a spider there is a chain of events the body undergoes before the visible reaction. The heart beats faster, and the breathing rate is also too high – the white blood cell count is increased. If you get injured in the forest, your body needs to fight off any infections that may result from a cut or bite – hospitals are far away.

A study showed that a chilly shower in the morning gives a stress response that allows the body to prepare for the day with increased white blood cell levels. The shower was warm but became cold in the last 30 seconds in one group; the other group kept the shower warm all the time. The body is kept free of infection. It was making the body better able to fight off any infection that may be hanging about.

The immune system can be boosted too much if there are too many aggressive neutrophils present. It will keep the immune cells in a high state of readiness when there is nothing to fight. A situation like this leads to problems, and one of the most common is allergies. According to Dr Ikharia, every allergy is because of an overactive immune system and the suffering is affected by fatigue because of the energy needed to maintain this state. This highly active state makes the system push it out of balance and can damage our health issues. Evidence shows that because our immune system is overworked, it cannot effectively fight off infections since it is overworked; tired.

Dr Mohamed Shamgi of Imperial College London deliberately provoked his immune system for science. He is allergic to grass pollen, house mites and cat hair; when exposed his body goes into a heightened state and histamine boosts blood flow to get white cells to the site; the skin goes red, we have an itchy nose and runny eyes. In the summer months, many of us stock up on antihistamines designed to reduce the release of the hormone into the bloodstream when the pollen count is high.

The number of people who suffer from allergies has increased worldwide, and it is down to a few reasons, including but not exclusive to junk food. A poor diet in diversity usually leads to low numbers of different gut bacteria that are important for immune cells to strive. Studies show that children that grow up in more rural environments, e.g., farms are more exposed to a wider variety of microbes that I explained elsewhere in this book. Contrastingly, children brought up in urban areas and kept indoors become more prone to allergic reactions. Without a cure for allergies, we must spend more time outdoors and eat a balanced diet not to develop the at all.

Exercising is sometimes overrated; this is because it has been monetised to within an inch of its life. However, it is no myth that a regular dose of moderate exercise up to five times per week can boost our immune systems five-fold according to some studies. The amount of activity is dependent on the individual; always talk to your health care professional before embarking on an exercise programme. Mobilising the cells around the body, moving lymphocytes to all areas with an increased heart rate at a level where you can talk but maybe not belt out a ballad is probably exactly right for the immune system.

Some evidence suggests that extreme exercise routines could leave you susceptible to infections, so a balanced, responsible approach is recommended. Massage is another little-known booster for the immune system; its effects on HIV is well documented - Professor Fluvio Acquisto, 2020, University of Roehampton, UK. He found that children who have AIDS responded to rounds of soft-touch therapy. Many more T-cells were produced, and he concluded that the same is true for all as touching and caressing is not only an emotional response.

These T- cells are brought to the surface of the skin, and they investigate to see if there are any invaders around. After a massage in an adult patient, it was recorded that not on were the lymphocyte T-cells increasing, but also other immune cells moved around looking for invaders. The professor suggests that the percentage increase could range between 10 and 23%, which is a fantastic number in immunity terms. He explained that there are nerves in the skin that connect to glands where T-cells are stored, and the rubbing of the skin causes the response that enables the increased levels of immune cells. In the context of the pandemic, massages are an excellent tool to help fight the disease.

Sleep is also a good indicator of how well the immune system will cope in a pandemic. To unmask corona is to look at several things we take for granted and our reliance on pharmaceuticals. All the areas I have covered in this chapter are ways in which the individual can responsibly look after themselves and those around them. The government must lead from the podium and bring society along with them; the messaging needs to be careful clear, concise, and consistent to obtain and maintain a constant internal environment in our God-given temple.

A vast army of immune cells are basophils, neutrophils, and macrophages; killer cells get to the frontline of an attack the invaders [fend off] – Team One all about speed and aggression. Sometimes invaders are swallowed whole, killed by chemicals or throw of nets to ensnare them, but sometimes it is not about the speed but rather the need for precision in defence.

Team Two – Lymphocyte T-cells and B-Cells, which are not as fast as first responders, but they are more effective in producing specific tools to mount specialised attacks with more devastating results - identifying invaders and preparing and carrying out custom-made attacks effectively and precisely. They provide protection from memory if an infection strikes

90

again. You may have known of or had the experience of certain infections and were told that you could only get it once; chickenpox is a typical example. This is described as long-term immunity. If all our immune cells are working well, they can repel attacks and eliminate threats quickly and efficiently, but when they struggle for whatever reason, that is when we become ill. So, yes, it is essential to have a fully functioning immune system to stay clear of disease.

How we strengthen and maintain a sound immune system is hotly debated. If you read the small print and the larger print too, almost every vitamin and mineral claims to boost immunity. One estimate is that over a billion pounds are spent in the UK annually on supplements, mostly with immunity in mind.

Professor Michael Heinrich [UCL, School of Pharmacy], states that Supplements help your immune system in a minor way [garlic and elderberry] is best taken in your food. Echinacea, however, is better as evidence shows that it prevents and in cases treats the common cold (some research suggests it could reduce the duration by almost a day and a half) and mild forms of influenza. We must be careful as some unscrupulous characters sell products that sometimes have none of the active ingredients of Echinacea in them; the Traditional Herbal Registration (THR) is the mark of authenticity for herbal products.

Vitamins and minerals are needed in small amounts, and we should be eating good quality food. Nutrients from citrus and red peppers are good [twice as rich in vitamins and minerals], cheese, meat and a wide range of seeds and nuts could provide enough zinc necessary for building new immune cells. There is evidence in studies that low levels of zinc can be attributed to COVID-19 cases according to a study by an institute in Barcelona, Spain. B vitamins provide energy for immune cells – peas, pulses, yoghurt, and seafood, especially mussels [one serving has seven times the required amount of B_{12}]. If the diet is balanced, then the need for supplements is reduced dramatically; conversely, if the plan is to compensate for a poor diet with a supplement, you are in trouble.

Vitamin D is essential, and the source is not always food, a daily 400 IU has been shown to increase disease-fighting cells. The immune cells are happiest and better at killing the bacteria and virus we come across when there is a sufficient level of this vitamin present. The quantity of sunlight is a talking point, and the answer is that the amount needed is dependent on pigmentation, the skin produces it. Research has shown that melanin slows down the production of vitamin D, so the darker your skin, the more sunlight needed to produce the same amount.

A rule of thumb is that a darker person needs to be exposed to sunlight 3 – 4 times longer than a lighter-skinned person to reap the same benefits - Professor Michael Heinrich UCL. Circumstances dictate how long you spend in the sun, during the UK's dark winter we struggle to get our full dosage so it is worthwhile using supplements (10 micrograms per day) throughout winter and many could benefit from having them all year round because of the intermittent nature of sunlight [Dr Ronx Ikharia; A&E]

Small lifestyle changes could enhance your immunity. Sleep, food, exercise, and a lack of stress are some of the things we can control. There is a lot to be gained from increasing foods rich in zinc as it has been proven to balance immune responses and have a direct antiviral action against viruses. I remember speaking to a medical doctor turned teacher who headed the biology department in a school I worked in the autumn of 2019 about flu symptoms. She had been working very hard during a difficult period where staff was frequently absent for various reasons and she was literally run off her feet. I will call her Dr KD, in the conversation to which I refer, she admitted to, feeling really rough the night before. When I asked why she bothered to turn up she said having taken zinc tablets the previous night she would be fine. I sought clarity on the matter and she explained the antiviral properties of zinc to me in some amount of detail.

Studies[7] from Europe, specifically Spain done during the first wave of the pandemic seem to indicate that it would be a great idea to continue to explore the role of this mineral. Another peer reviewed study from Asia; India in particular, showed that there is an increased level of zinc had an immune-regulatory compound. A different, significant finding was that patients with zinc deficiency displayed a higher level of mortality than those with better levels of zinc.

Chapter 3

Past, Present and Future...
World without end...

Character is destiny; it matters in government... In 1998 America was booming after the end of the cold war, it was a great time to be in America. Prosperity was much more under the Bush or Obama's administration. Then, President Bill Clinton was morally deficient. He had that affair with Monica Lewinsky, lied about it, and tried to obstruct justice by lying under oath.

It was the case that the conservative White Evangelical movement, including Southern Baptists, sanctioned high political office standards. They introduced that resolution tied to scripture and profound theological truth in which one of the clauses said: 'tolerance of serious wrong by public office holders scorched the decency of a culture and seeds immortality and will result in God's judgment'. This was embraced by the American evangelical crusaders of the day; they cheered it to the rafters.

94

Did we see the reawakening of white evangelicalism during the last four years in the USA? Trump walking out and about without a mask in the White house's grounds, without a mask at the height of a pandemic, is a stark reminder. Before Reagan, American evangelicals were not keen on politics until the moral majority movement (Jerry Falwell) took root before he came to power. By the time of Reagan's reign, politics through the republican door was in bed with evangelicals.

They are certainly far from silent in their rallying to president, Donald Trump, whose personal traits make him a completely improbable vessel for evangelical aspirations: three times married, accused in a manner credible multiple extramarital affairs, ready to speak vulgarly. He talked about grabbing women by the genitals, demeaning immigrants from developing countries and said, in defiance of a central Christian tenet, that he has never seen any reason to ask God for forgiveness

Fast forward a couple of decades and the decay could not be more evident. If the polls now are anything to go by, they show that the group least likely to stand on the premise that character matters would be white evangelicals. They sacrificed truth on the altar of partisanship; core truths did not matter to them anymore. Conservative Christian evangelicals used the power of Christianity to usher in the most repulsive, unashamedly cruel, ignorant, lying, and incompetent, morally bankrupt, hardnosed, intolerant of many of his fellow citizens named Donald J. Trump into the most powerful political office in the world, the White House.

Chapter 3

Trump is escorted into the White House by the wind of support of these same Christians, this faction that previously embraced the idea that character is destiny. When it was time for these people to stand up and be counted, they sacrificed. The pandemic caused many world leaders to despair; he carelessly communicated to the people of America, arrogantly telling them that it was nothing to worry about. Even when he knew better because the world had warned him, he casually said that the fifteen or so cases that were reported in America would soon be down to zero. The American people and by extension, the world had been misled by the president. When his people and the world required strong leadership with direct and clear messaging at the beginning of the pandemic, he spewed confusion, oozed incompetence, and tweeted on and on...

Past president Donald Trump was so careless in his approach that when George Floyd was killed, and his people rose over centuries of pain his reaction was that of a pyromaniac pouring fuel on the flames of discontent and racial upheaval due to deep-rooted divisions. He watched his police force assault peaceful protesters, cleared out priests from their own churches so he could play on the 'conscience' of his people by standing in front of a church and waving a bible in the air symbolising something different from what his life represented.

The world experiencing the fruits of a great con and he is doing all the things he said he would not do, there is hatred at an unprecedented height a divided nation and the lying and cruelty keeps coming. The choice of leader the white conservative evangelical churches' candidate of choice is everything but what the church was founded on and is where it should stand.

The mask of the corona pandemic is not enough to cover the scabs of the deep wounds of racism and inequality that have been torn open in the 'Trumpian' era in America.

Approximately, a quarter of a million Americans, over a hundred and thirty thousand in the UK and over a million worldwide have died from the virus to date. The principles of love and to exhibit the fruits of the spirit are the standards on which we Christians should live.

He surrounded himself with people like Stephen Bannan who called for the beheading of Dr Anthony Fauci and Christopher Wray, the FBI director... Bannan was not banned from Facebook, and CEO, Mark Zuckerberg justified to congress why the company did not take down his account. The social media platform saw sense in removing the video even though it was after about ten hours. Zuckerberg told his staff that Bannan had 'not violated enough policies to justify a ban' (Guardian 13/11/2020).

The paper reported that Twitter had permanently banned the podcast called War Room that Bannan was using to spout his hate, giving the reason as; 'the podcast account violated its policy on the glorification of violence'. If this were an Islamist, there would be no hesitation to remove the account and lean on the perpetrator, or would there? The long arm of the US law would be extending into the far reaches of wherever these dissidents were hiding.

The mind boggles at the anger and hatred displayed by people dying from COVID -19, the denial is unreal - they do not want their families or loved ones to be called when their oxygen levels suggest death is on the horizon. They refuse the nurses' requests to contact them, saying that the situation cannot be real, and it will be all right. These scenarios seen all over America are symptomatic of what the people have assimilated based on the diet fed to them by the president. When he took ill before the elections and then flaunted the medical protocols, he was called out by members of his medical team for risking other people's lives and livelihood.

The then president in a limousine trip on the campaign trail waved and removed his mask, which was seen as heroic to some of his supporters; he reveled in it as the world watched. The storming of the United States Capitol on January 6th, 2021 did not happen out of the blue. It happened because of a forty-year programme of pressing and crushing spirits, coming to a head when the latest installment of a president in the most extensive 'democracy in the world' came down.

Frank Schaeffer, an ex-Orthodox Christianity convert, poured his heart out on social media claiming that he was responsible in no small way for the awful situation in the United States. He was responding to the ugly scenes we saw in Washington, D.C. He made one very telling point that white evangelicals, of whom he was an active part as a young white fanatic, were responsible.

Frank said that he is now and has been 'a liberal activist who mostly voted for the Democratic Party' for a long time. He mentioned the role of his father Francis Schaeffer, in his last book 'A Christian manifesto', the United States Government's violent overthrow. He is reported to have said that if 'Roe v. Wade wasn't reversed, and abortion made illegal by democratic means the Americans had a right to revolution' (Francis Schaeffer – A Christian manifesto). He is mainly accountable for 'striking the match that lit the fire that started' the Religious Right of America on its current course to 'take back America for God.' The evangelicals were at the forefront of the attack on the USA parliament building; they were the children and grandchildren of people whom Schaeffer influenced all those years ago. Schaeffer writes the following hard hitting statement in his book. 'What we must understand is that the two world views really do bring forth with inevitable certainty not only personal differences in regard to society, government, and law. There is no way to mix two total world views'. The Schaeffer's were responsible for a nepotistic reign of theocratic terror on the USA according to Frank. He fingered players in this deadly game, some of whom I mentioned rallied around the Ronald Reagan administration all those years ago.

It is the feeling of many that the election and mainstay of support for the preceding US president comes from this demography. Franklin Graham from the Billy Graham empire and Ralph Reid a political operative is credited with making Donald Trump, president. Reid is a serial fundraiser for the movement – evangelical. There is not a political problem as we know it in the USA, according to Frank Schaeffer.

He didn't like the official melding of church and state, but his exhortation to readers was that Christianity, properly applied, brings forth not only certain personal results, but also governmental and legal results. Schaeffer's big point was that, for too long, American Christians had divided the world into spiritual and material spheres, and that they had applied Christianity only to the former. Schaeffer taught that 'the Lordship of Christ covers *all* of life and *all* of life equally.' However, instead, there is a religious fanaticism problem akin to what we see in Iran, only this one is Christian.

Without the evangelical movement, churches, pastors, newsletters radio hosts and authors like Stephen Strang (God, Trump and COVID) going along with the president's rhetorical half-truths and outright lies, who supported him into the White House, he would not have been there.

America has been in a war of religion where white fundamentalist evangelicals and their conservative Roman Catholic allies have squared off against American democracy because they are out to create a theocracy – '… a bigoted evangelical version of Iran' – (Frank Schaeffer 2021). Schaeffer believed Christians needed to follow a path of *escalating* actions, and he left no doubt where those actions led if they were not successful. The seventies and eighties saw the birth of all this according to sources.

American democracy is on life support, and it has not gone unnoticed by Russia, Iran, China, and the like. The media is not blameless in the debacle; mainstream and social. They talk about the Russ Belt, and poor working-class Americans in dire straits, all true, but the elephant in the room isn't covered. White evangelicals do not get the coverage; some say that is because they are providing the content… they are afraid to get into the truth about the white nationalist and the racist movement in which it has morphed.

Frank Schaeffer opines that the 'theology is a myth; stuff evangelicals believe in is a myth; it did not happen. What they do not believe in actually happened.' He gives examples of science, global warming, and democracy; all are happening and do happen. In his tirade, Schaeffer echoed my thoughts that America who regularly went into countries worldwide and meddled in their internal affairs was the laughingstock of those autocratic regimes; citing it as proof that America is failing. The previous president was capable and undoubtedly did incalculable damage to the USA before he eventually leaves office. He has presided over the party that debased debate over feminism, gender, and race, and has gone after women and people of other sexual orientations.

A litany of atrocities culminated in the 2020 killings of people like Michael Brown, Brianna Taylor, George Floyd, and several black people killed by law enforcement officers between 2017 and 2020. Statista recorded these mind-blowing numbers; a total of 3986 deaths over the period, 893 were blacks and 643 were Hispanics, making up 38.48% of all killings by law enforcement.

Recently, ever since the shooting of Michael Brown in 2014 in Missouri, police homicides drew comparisons between police in the USA and countries like England that had much lower numbers. The Black Lives matter also brought more attention to the frequency and number of civilians shot by police.

Chapter 3

(Statista;https://www.statista.com/statistics/585152/people-shot-to-death-by-us-police-by-race/)

The party of theocracy [the Republican Party] backed groups in

Number of people shot to death by the police in the United States from 2017 to 2021, by race

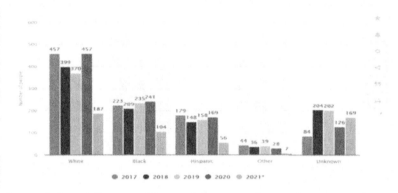

USA spitting bile, conflicts of interest is at the root of the problem. That is the reason they are so up in arms about the amendment giving them the right to bear arms; that may be why the National Rifle Association (NRA) are seen as untouchables by some. The courts are stacked with bible-beating evangelicals who want the country to be democratic but ruled by the theocrats who wish to impose their brand of morality on the nation's people.

India is a case in point as it relates to society's need to accept shared responsibility; the pandemic and all the negative connotations. I am devastated by what I will write about for the remainder of this chapter because it brings to light a very disgraceful plight that girls and women in India face.

102

Period emergency in India... the parents do not know what the menstruation period is about. There are few toilet facilities in some places in India, there are two for hundreds of girls and the teachers. Their government hand out sanitary products and many have resorted to cloth and other very poor alternatives. Discrimination against menstruating women is widespread in India, where periods have long been a taboo and considered impure.

Societally, they have been excluded from events, denied entry to temples and shrines and, believe it or not, kept out of kitchens. There is a World Menstrual Hygiene day which takes place on May 28th each year. It has been documented that due to the lack of conversation around the issue, 71% of adolescent girls in India are unaware of menstruation until they get it themselves according to one study.

One BBC News report claims that campaigners say it shows that parents rarely prepare their daughters for something they know is bound to unfold. The lack of preparation leads to much inescapable fear and anxiety. It is a major difficulty of getting sanitary pads is another big problem. The tax on these products was scrapped; it was at 12% up until 2018 following campaigns.

The reported study revealed that 36% of the women of menstruating age used sanitary napkins, with the others using old rags, ash, leaves, mud, husk and soil. It beggars belief as the level of risk associated with this practice of stemming the blow flow during this period.

Chapter 3

The coronavirus pandemic has made matters much worse according to health experts in the country. Lockdown severely affected the reduction and supply of menstrual products. It is essential to note that period poverty does not only affect the women in India but many more stakeholders are impacted.

The international community is heavily involved and charity called Plan International UK stated that one in 10 disadvantaged girls below the age of 21 are not able to afford sanitary napkins and uses very unhygienic alternatives such as newspapers, toilet paper and even socks.

Very early in an Indian girl's life, the fear and severe pain set in. They learn to live with the lack of help with the physical and mental trauma associated with their period, something westerners take for granted. Social media; in the recent past females have shared stories that were previously hidden in taboo and myth, previously masked by culture and tradition.

That did not fully liberate the women as they still suffered the wrath of those not wanting their stories to be aired. That resulted in the threat of bans while those who trolled and shamed the women were never punished. Calls are to give these women a voice and not to shame and stigmatise them, but to instead give them knowledge and freedom to deal with their trauma. Social media is a powerful tool that should be used to amplify awareness among the population.

Chapter 4

Spirituality vs. the Ego

Approaching the matter of spirituality, we think of godly elements: tolerance, love, forgiveness and a humble lifestyle. We don't normally think of ego. In fact, one often joins the spiritual path to become free from ego. Unfortunately, sometimes you meet your shadow on the exact road you took to avoid it[1].

The real danger is not COVID-19; it is the battle for the hearts and minds of the people. We need to guard our minds against offense; it is the foundation of the strategy the enemy is using to conquer the heats of the nations. There is a movement where the world is awash by a storm of offense; the brethren are accused, engulfed by slander, gossip, and offense. One of the world's biggest problems in our world today is the trap set for believers and non-believers in the form of offense.

Does it matter that some people struggle to understand that real spirituality is not about being better or being on a higher level than others. Eventually, some people's spiritual ego blinded them to their own behavior and how their spiritual progress was making them act around others.

A quotation from the late Buddhist Chogyam Trungpa Rinpoche reads:

Chapter 4

"There are numerous sidetracks which lead to a distorted, ego-centered version of spirituality; we can deceive ourselves into thinking we are developing spirituality when instead we are strengthening our egocentricity through spiritual techniques. This fundamental distortion may be referred to as spiritual materialism."

If I'd read that full of spiritual ego I would have thought I was lucky not to be that person. Some many individuals are caught up in the grip of spiritual narcissism and spiritual egotism.

In areas of the world like Thailand with a rich heritage of spiritual development in today's society have some amazing people. The reality of how overpowering spiritual ego can get now it can create this self-perpetuating industry of 'being woke' has been a sight to see.

People are so easily offended that the smallest of thing cause us to lose tempers, get into scraps, lash out and even take the lives of others. We are to try and stop the spread of the virus that is offense and SARS-CoV-2 is nowhere near as infectious as the storm that is blowing in the lives of the people of the world today. In his letters to Timothy (*2 Timothy 3:1-17*), Paul outlines to the young pastor that things will worsen. He emphasises that times will become harder, especially for people who were lovers of themselves.

Self-love is a good thing in so far as it is not the reason for which we live. We must seek shelter in the one who created us; Psalm 91 provides solace – "Whoever *dwells in the shelter of the Most High will rest in the shadow of the Almighty"* [2](NIV).

106

Humanity has always sought to satisfy its lusts more than to please the creator and do as He had directed. In a world where man is more zealous to grab what he can to obtain and genuinely concerned to maintain what he has made, makes him very treacherous to his fellow human beings.

The gospel is not taken seriously in today's world for a number of reasons including but not limited to man (mankind) losing the fear of God. He has lost the obedience as children are disobedient to their parents. Nations have become consumed with the lust for power at all costs just as the Bible warned. Times are perilous, unholy men have lost the fear of God, and the mercies are taken for granted.

We must separate the truth from half-truths and blatant lies... Dr. Martin Luther King was not popular in the black church community until he was dead, he was in the South with Jesse Jackson, but the North had nothing to do with him. He became the Southern Christian Leadership Conference (SCLC) leader roundabout 1955 after he led the Montgomery bus boycott and subsequently led other movements, some of which failed[3].

There has been disconnection between Africa and African Americans, a difference between the living word on Sunday and what happens in our lives from Monday to Saturday. Kelly Brown Douglas said, "We can't talk about homosexuality because we can't talk about sexuality"[5]. She cited that a recent pew study indicated that the Black Church community was more opposed to these issues than other communities. The study cited 64 percent of African Americans opposing same sex marriages, a percentage that held steady for several years, while the overall population had become less opposed to those marriages (from 41 percent in 1996 to 20 percent in 2003).[6]

The experience of the black family shaped the black preaching in the South. Many were products of a society in the segregated Carolinas where the black child was not to become literate; the ability to read or write. The climate pervaded with racist thought, racist teaching and racist practices. It was even against the law to introduce an African to reading. Northern white missionaries came to the schools to teach the schools to set up 'hybridism' in the early 1900s.

European and British culture introduced as being synonymous with Christianity, hybridism. Female Preachers, even though well-educated and experienced in the 1940s, 50s and 60s were not called preachers but instead called Ministers, or Women's day speakers.

One of Donald Trump's advisors, Pastor Mark Burns spoke to Ian Dale on LBC and openly lobbied for Trump on the night of the election stating that the people had a champion in the White House, and he would have been re-elected to office in the November elections of 2020. He talked about Roe v. Wade and how black lives did not matter (reference to the protests of summer 2020) if unborn babies do not matter.

He presented a differing view on the life of Jesus and how he handled matters presented before him. Christian ministers have made videos about how Donald Trump would retain the office of president. The Bible talks about the idea of leadership throughout. Jeremiah spoke to leaders in a general sense; he addressed: political leaders, business leaders, military leaders, education leaders, and spiritual leaders. David Guzik points out "In our day, we could put the first emphasis about pastors as spiritual leaders." My view is that we need servant leaders.

Scripture records, the flock of Jeremiah's day, were effectively dispersed. Some taken away to Babylon and other nations as prisoners, and others went as refugees to Egypt. We can trace all this back to ungodly and wretched leaders for the people of God; we are told that John in 1 John: 12 (NLT) that we must be careful and not listen to all those who claim to be from God. John said, "Dear friends, do not think that all those who claim to speak by the Spirit, you must test them to see if the Spirit has come from God, for there are many false prophets in the world."[7]

Christians are called to be aware of anyone claiming to be a prophet who falsely claims to speak in the name of God, or the name of another god must die (Deuteronomy 18:20 -22); to Christians ,usually, God told them different things. The question should be asked if they are ready for the message delivered. If the said prophecy does not come through as prophesied, then the prophet must not be referenced, supported, or feared.

It was Jeremiah who said, "I heard these prophets say, 'Listen to the dream I had from God last night', and then they proceed to tell lies in my name. How long will this go on? If they are prophets of deceit, inventing everything they say. By telling these false dreams, they are trying to get my people to forget me, just as their ancestors did by worshipping the idols of Baal" (Jeremiah 23:25-28).

People are so mired in self that they seek to appear so deep in their faith, being so connected that God singles them out for service. Jeremiah declares falsehood from the "dreams" of these prophets is allowed. However, true messengers should faithfully proclaim the Word. He points out that the difference will be as transparent as that between "straw and grain!".

Apostle Gino Jennings postulated that the liars were so loyal to Donald Trump's re-election into the White House that 'these heathens and white evangelicals lied to God' (*Deuteronomy 18, Jeremiah 23:24*). A number of these false prophets have recorded themselves or posted on social media racking up tens of thousands of views, likes and shares leading up to the American election of 2020.

Chris Hume is a case in point; it is a shocking revelation of the number of 'sheep' that follow these charlatans. "The Lord has anointed and appointed Donald Trump to be the next president of the USA." Hume claimed. He had given lots of prophecies and dreams before and he should be held responsible for what happened on the day of the presidential inauguration.

The man was so certain of himself that he gave the proviso that no one should jump to conclusions and continued to defend what he heard from the Lord even as the evidence overwhelmed him that Trump had lost. As Christ-followers, we must desist from validating these claims by liking and commenting on the videos.

I have mentioned that Pat Robertson, Robin Bullock spoke to the Lord, received the negative response, and Kevin Zadai was guaranteed a second term for Trump. Michelle Bachmann saw the result sealed by God, Tracey Cooke, Kat Kerr said Trump would sit in that office for four more years. "God will have his way in this country" was echoed by this band of evangelicals.

Pastor Denise Goulet – International Church of Las Vegas, Robert Henderson saw several dreams. In the third he said he was selected as a running mate for Trump in his second term, Hank Kuneman saw two terms for the "one from New York". Kent Christmas, Mark Taylor were convinced, Greg Locke with "full complete assurance and opinionated authority Donald Trump won by a landslide", Terri Pearsons prayed that Trump would triumph by any means necessary to "Bring it all in line! Bring it all in line; get it all in line with the will of God!" Lance Willinau prayed for the angel of the Lord to go forth because the president can't fight, Paula White with her spiritual insight spoke in tongues as I have mentioned.

She was calling on spirits from Africa and South America, etc. Kurt Landry called for prayers for Trump the swing states would go red for Trump. In this book, Kenneth Copland has been mentioned and they used their offices to ridicule God in the election's run-up and aftermath.

Marcus Rodgers, another of the prophets who continued to tell the world about his dreams. God gave him a revelation that he could not interpret, but he knows that "Trump will be president and something big is coming…" - The Beat by Allen Parr[3]. **(Jeremiah 23:30 -32)** Repentance is a thing of beauty; Kris

111

Valloton, a Bethel Church pastor, came online and congratulated the incoming president and then proceeded to apologise for 'missing the prophecy'.

Funny, though; he appears to have a change of heart, and the statement removed shortly afterwards. He called it right for Trump in 2016 and later prophesied that Trump would not be impeached and returned for a second term. That has not happened, and he is claiming not to be a false prophet but is sorry to have let down those who trusted in him. I think he should be reading from Jeremiah 23:26 until he gets it right.

Sid Roth took to Facebook live to bring the world up to respond to the election and prophesies. It's beggar's belief that the man publicly declared that the deposed president was the first president in his lifetime and fifty years of ministry to be so decorated. He was a) Pro-life, the first to attend a pro-life rally, b) Pro–Israel since Harry Truman and c) the most Judaeo-Christian, pro-religious freedom president.

Sid could not understand how Trump did not win the second term in office; he apologised and took full responsibility for what he said. He was disappointed for those of us whose faith faltered when we heard he would win and did not.

This man is on the record talking about the Jewish people and trumpeted the mantra "the Trump's economic policies were successful because of his love for Israel." Roth used 1 Corinthians 4:5 to talk about the great things on the cards for America, 'Golden Global Glory' God will do exceedingly, abundantly above all that we can ask or think. His apolitical upbringing has not prevented him being a Republican Jewish evangelist who believes "the Devil has overplayed his hand". Sid is making a case for the false prophesy that we witnessed by mentioning Jonah and his message for Nineveh; the city escaped destruction not destroyed immediately but two centuries later.

There is a battle going on with Christians worldwide. Habakkuk called on God, questioned God about the state of the world (Habakkuk 1:1 - 4, 11) during his time and received an answer he found difficult to accept (v. 12 – 17), but God knew better and had another plan. It is the will of God for all to be saved; Isaiah 60:1-3 speaks about the gentiles (non-Jews) rising and blessing Zion.

There will be a reshaping of the church, Israel, the USA, and the world; it will be filled with glory. Restoration will return to the earth, and the fear of the Lord will return; no man will be credited for the recognition, a forever glory and unbelievers will be overwhelmed for God will be glorified forever.

Republicans were duped; the elections were not stolen. A Trump statement at the time was; the election was "corrupt" and "was indeed the big lie."The facts are, no widespread corruption was discovered and nothing was stolen from Trump. The labeling of every peaceful protest as anything but...

Antifa is a group of antifascists fighting against the ills of Trumpism led by a perfect cult leader who put a smile on the faces of the remainder of the world that are enemies of American democracy. During the Trump years this movement gained mythical status, labeled by the former USA president and those supporting them as terrorists according to a Reuters report. White evangelicals and other white nationalists elected a man who was about nothing or anyone but himself.

His messaging became the fuel poured on the flames of lies and led people to believe that Democrats were Satan worshipping, child killers and paedophiles who stole their country. His supporters were so much on edge, wound up that they prepared for months before the election, some held up in bushes with heavy artillery performing mock battles in preparation for the country's defense. They were willing to die for their leader, culminating with the most significant terror attack on America since the horrors of 9/11.

There is obviously a battle between the opposing forces in play in our world, each pulling in opposite directions. Are we spiritual beings? Both material and divine; the ego according to psychologists and theorists plays a critical role in the human psyche. According to Madonna "I am a material girl, living in a material world". The physical brain made from material is the source of human consciousness.

Essentially, the ego shapes what-makes-us who we are and spirituality is that which has its focus beyond the material world. When we look past the material [a lot of religious people are materialistic] the concept of our identity considerably increases. The reality of what-makes-us-us is not the thoughts of us swirling around in our brain, but instead is the vast awareness behind the thoughts. We are not beliefs and thoughts but rather part of a greater entirety…

114

Chapter 5

I beg your pardon.

'Why?' This is a question frequently asked by people, from toddlers to grand mamas and papas. It is one of the first questions asked by toddlers, especially, and this continues throughout life. The most extensive use of the word may be about God and the Bible. An example may have been 'Why did Jesus leave heaven and come to earth in the flesh?' or, 'Why do people act in defiance of the authority set up to keep everything and everyone safe?'

Men and women have written volumes on the subject, trying to answer the question. It is possible to partly answer that the Old Testament said that God would become incarnate on earth. What that means is, if Jesus had not been born as a Messiah Man, the prophets like Isaiah would be wrong.

The Bible records hundreds of predictions in the Old Testament concerning the First Initiation of Jesus Christ. All fulfilled by Him during His time on earth. Interestingly Jesus himself told His disciples the Law, the Prophets and the Psalms all spoke about His arrival. They were on point; he came and delivered according to the promise. Isaiah declared the reason why Jesus came; he prophesied that Jesus came to keep God's promise to send a Saviour into the world - *Isaiah 9:6 -7*.

Chapter 5

We go from the good word of the bible to the dastardly ways of politics...

The USA constitution Article II, section 2[1] gives the president power to pardon people guilty of transgressing the law of the land. Interestingly, President Donald Trump was busy over the Christmas period wielding his presidential pen in explaining to several of his loyalists as he prepared to demit the office he had held onto for four years. Different States also have the autonomy to pardon those who violated state laws[2].

It is usual for the application for pardon to be addressed to the president directly. A pardon by the constitution can only be granted when the request is an admission of guilt on the part of the seeker of the pardon[3]. It is often the case that some applicants are not given this pardon because they have not accepted responsibility. Donald Trump had thrown the congress in the United States into mayhem with Roger Jason Stone's clearing, a loyalist who let a police dog go on a man. He was infamous from the late 1970s as a dirty trickster whilst working with the Young Republicans Organisation[4].

Another pardon went to one from that same era known as Paul Manafort; hired by Trump and described as one of his many unethical political cronies. Manafort was hired in 2016 to run the campaign machinery, and we were all sceptical after learning that his recent job before that was a political strategist for a Ukrainian dictator[5]. It stood to reason because Manafort had made his money helping despots and would-be despots parade as legitimate, making him a symbol of the political system's corruption. Ronald Reagan employed these two to run his campaign in the North-East and the South when he ran for office[5].

Manafort held several critical positions in the republican organisation and was one of the principal fundraisers, who had money pouring in. He was a money-grabbing man who would stop at nothing to be near a lot of it. The firm 'Manafort, Black and Stone' was formed when Stone and Manafort decided to monetise their influence in political circles and hired Lee Atwater known as the grandfather of negative politics.

They offered political consulting along with other traditional promoting and obtained a significant advantage over their rivals. They were a syndicate akin to football agents, incidentally, working for all three Republican candidates in the 1988 elections. When a candidate they backed gained power, they gained access and influence.

Manafort may have secrets for Donald Trump; he refused to testify when asked. His loyalty to Donald Trump was impregnable, and he got pardoned as a result. 'Political corruption continues to be rife; the unfettered influence of megabucks, the prominence of a lobbyist at the top of the political pyramid, tax havens and interference in elections by foreign powers makes it inevitable for the president's ability to pardon to be managed' [6] *thehill.com.*

Booming Biopharmaceuticals…

Therapeutics and biopharmaceutical companies are popping up all around the world from Israel to Britain to the United States. They are specialising in the development of patient-oriented targeted therapy for many diseases, including cancers. The research and development lead to scientists identifying conditions much more quickly, and therefore treatments will be more available. Even investors in the stock market predict that the next five years' biggest movers will be in the genomic space - *Cathy Wood – ARK Invest*.

She singled out DNA sequencing, artificial intelligence, and gene therapies among massive growth areas to watch as the convergence would cure diseases, even diabetes, which draws the most considerable portion of the healthcare budget of most western economies[7].

She rightly asserts that we now have real science and technology surfacing and suggested that the mutations in our genomic profiles, exposing the disease's earliest manifestations. There is no question in my mind that people must display much discipline; responsible behaviour must be stressed; the more transmission there is the more mutations. We know from science that with each modification, the chance of the virus changing significantly increases, making vaccines lose their efficiency greater.

The Bible bears several accounts of healing, especially during the time of Jesus. *Revelation 21:14* boldly states that this will come to pass; '*He will wipe every tear from their eyes, there will be no more death or mourning or crying or pain, for the old order of things has passed away*'[8].

Mark 5:34 '*He said to her, "Daughter, your faith has healed you. Go in peace and be freed from your suffering."*'[9]

Psalm 103:1-5 *'Praise the Lord, my soul; all my inmost being, praise his holy name. Praise the Lord, my soul, and forget not all his benefits – who forgives all your sins and heals your diseases, who redeems your life from the pit and crowns you with love and compassion, who satisfies your desires with good things so that your youth is renewed like the eagle's'[10].*

Matthew 4:23 (NIV) *'Jesus went through Galilee, teaching in their synagogues, proclaiming the good news of the kingdom, and healing every disease and sickness among the people.'[11]*

Healthcare has been in the news, and even the money markets are getting filled with companies concentrating on conditions that have bled economies of most countries for decades. Companies are working in Genome-editing technology areas since only a small percentage of monogenic diseases have any treatments today[12]. The symptoms of conditions are being treated, and the underlying root causes of diseases are ignored or remain evasive.

Responsible companies have embarked upon using cutting-edge technology that will help to edit genes simply and economically. Genes can be corrected, repaired, or deleted with precision. Diseases like: cystic fibrosis, childhood blindness, Thalassemia, cancers, and sickle cell anemia are a few of the thousands of conditions that make life difficult for humankind – CRISPR /Cas9. CRISPR is on track to be the first company to offer a cure for Thalassemia according to the positive data shown up to 80% gene modification with no off-target editing[13].

Chapter 5

CRX1 will be a single dose curative therapy for patients suffering from Thalassemia and severe sickle cell anemia. The Genomics Age and less than twenty years after its introduction, a human genome's cost has fallen to less than six thousand United States dollars. Research suggests it should be fewer than one hundred in the next five years driving the genomic sequencing[14].

We are fighting the giant of fear in our lives

I think of those people, known and unknown to me whose thoughts are bothered, and anxiety rocks them whether because of difficult circumstances or poor mental health. Lord, I pray you will draw near to them even when they find it challenging to remove near you...

It is an unleavened diet of fear that is fed to the populations of the world during this pandemic. Media houses and social media are awash with memes, lies, misinformation and disinformation. Doctors and clinicians all signatories of the 'Great Barrington Declaration'[15] promoting 'focused protection' which said that people without underlying medical conditions would not be harmed by returning to everyday life. It was supposed to enable the population to acquire herd immunity[16].

The declaration was swiftly deemed inauthentic, as unethical, and fantastic by professors, researchers, scientists, and other health officials globally. It was unworkable, and as rumour had it, the actual document was not secure and could have anyone

120

as a signatory. There was a report of name fakers including 'Dr Johnny Bananas'.

Doctors from prestigious institutions drafted the declaration; Dr Sunetra Gupta of Oxford University, Dr Jay Bhattacharya of Stanford University, and Martin Kulldorff of Harvard University. They encountered the lack of peer-reviewed studies about SARS-CoV-2 and even asked policy decision makers to rely on 'herd immunity'. This is an idea that many, including prominent politicians like Boris Johnson and Donald Trump having limited knowledge of the subject, were convinced by epidemiologists without real data.

Trump was confident that the disease was 'not a big threat' and this gave oxygen to the opponents of lockdowns and citing the economic impact as a reason to avoid locking down earlier than they did [17].After a four-day conference in America, people told a Libertarian think tank – American Institute for Economic Research[18].

They should 'go back to living normally, practicing simple hygiene and staying home when they were sick'; this intimated that there was no need for face masks or social distancing[19]. The Facebook post that carried that 'breaking news' being flagged as dubious and inaccurate.

Change your perspective and look at another angle, the story surrounding the disproportionate number of Black and ethnic minority (BAME) people suffering and dying from the pandemic. We have been fed stories of healthcare workers and the ordinary 'Jill' and 'Joe' affected significantly more by the virus globally, particularly in the UK and USA. The reasons are many and varied, so it is prudent that we do not get carried away by the waves of doubt and fear culminating in a tsunami of conspiracy theories.

We must always be responsible in our reading, listening, and watching of content produced by sensationalists and the conversations we become involved in every step of our life's journey, but now even more so. It has never been more important to filter what we internalise. The remedies that have stood the test of time, the bush/bush grandma used to boil for pretty much any complaint cannot be just casted aside. There should be no room for cohesion on any side of this mutli-pronged argument, people must be allowed the right to decide what they put into their bodies…

Anecdotally, the American vaccination programme has issues around manufacturing, distribution and the stubborn number of Americans who are resisting the vaccination, citing different reasons including ethnicity. The centre for disease control (CDC) has used the science and the scientists to try and convince the doubters. The profile of a young 34 yrs. old black viral immunologist named Kizzmekia Corbett from a humble background was one attempt to help temper vaccine hesitancy[20]. She explained how the vaccine development process unfolded from the start of the programme just over a year before.

She led the team of doctors who were able to brief the then USA president and his task force on the work done on the Moderna vaccine as early as March last year. She said "The vaccine teaches the body to identify the spike protein, and the body identifies it and goes to work fighting against it..." She did not realise how much impact her presence had. She had done her work because of her love for science.

Corbett attended the University of Maryland, Baltimore County on a Meyerhoff Scholars Program – an aggressive programme for black minorities and women in America, the same alma mater as the Surgeon General, Jerome Adams, another black man. Statistics are that only 18% of all students graduate with a STEM degree, and only 2% are black. She was a people person, and good at science from an early age; the University spotted that fact–*Dr Freeman Hrabowski,* University president. The University is aware of the need for the population to see medics and scientists generally representing their demography. In the case of the vaccination programme thought, it engenders trust.

The Trust Factor explained considering he grew up in Birmingham hearing the Tuskegee University sanctioned experiment to see the long-term effects of syphilis on black men by letting it go untreated[18] – Guinea pigs. In the USA at the time and even since the COVID-19 has affected Native Americans, Black and Latino Americans at a much higher rate than it did others. Some of the reasons provided for this included racism and historical segregation.

Another example is Henrietta Lack's case, whose cancer cells were taken without her permission and used in billion-dollar medical studies without compensation[19]. Hrabowski said it is a painful truth that supposedly 'objective' scientists cared about

Chapter 5

everyone but valued people of colour less. His opinion was that Dr Corbett's authenticity showed the small-town upbringing and her Christian faith. The hope is that her story will cut through and appease the masses of 'ethnics' yet still be convinced.

She was aware of the issues facing the population; *Dr Anthony Fauci* praised her and used her credentials to plug the Moderna vaccine to the sceptics; he told the people of the USA "...the vaccine you're about to take was developed by an African American woman."[20] Dr Hrabowski even ended an interview saying that she must be the way forward as she showed people of all persuasions what was possible; "little girls needed to see her..."[21] .He explained that society does not give opportunities to gifted young people; the youngest 'freshman' he ever had was aged 9. His university would regularly earn their first degree by age 13 years old.- (**CBS, this morning**)

Institutional racism is a 'thing' but not in this case... There are the stop and search issues, and black women die five times more regularly from childbirth than their white counterparts. Faith plays a role in the community is resistant to the vaccine – cultural remedies have now become widely accepted after being demonised. A sense of mistrust is born, and the people you demonised are now being called on to be part of the system that fixes this mess – vaccine hesitancy.

Religion, language and even the media have conspired to make the job of the messengers much more difficult. The context is justifiable, but a case in point requires rational thinking,

124

something that has been absent from the psyche of people of colour for generations.

Government looks like they are not coherent in their approach to the pandemic, which feeds into the narrative that social media messages bring to the populace so efficiently and effectively. After the Black Lives Matter (BLM) protest of 2020, the government of the UK, headed by Boris Johnson commissioned a review into Race and Ethical Disparities headed by the controversial Dr Tony Sewell, a black educational consultant.

Sewell had previously suggested that evidence for institutional racism in the UK was 'somewhat flimsy' and as such when the report came out at the end of March 2021; it drew criticism from all corners of the society. The former teacher who worked with Prime minister on the Education Inquiry panel when Johnson was Mayor of London was not received whole-heartedly when he was appointed in June of 2020 and the Muslim council of Britain complained then that Dr. Sewell was not a convert and was 'keen on downplaying race disparities'.

Windrush expendable presence...

[1] The Guardian: I've been here for 50 years: the scandal of the former Commonwealth citizens threatened with deportation

[2] The Guardian: Windrush: two years on, victims describe long waits and 'abysmal' payouts

[3] The Independent: Hundreds of Windrush victims still waiting as only 1 percent of compensation is paid

Chapter 5

The Independent: Nine out of ten Wind rush applicants still waiting for compensation payouts

[4] The Independent: 'Hostile environment' broke law and is 'shameful stain on British history', equality watchdog finds

The Guardian: Home Office broke equalities law with hostile environment measures

[5] See note [4]

[6] 38 Degrees: Windrush: never again petition

[7] The Guardian: Black official quit 'racist' Windrush compensation scheme

[8] The Independent: Black official quits 'racist' Windrush compensation scheme over its failure to help victims

However, the vaccine has been rolled out to everyone's response to the prejudices in the shadows leading up to the pandemic. Unmasking corona is a way of looking at the mistreatment suffered by the people expected to be part of the solution to a pandemic. We must listen to what most people's objections to the vaccination are and then try to point out that we protect ourselves and those around us if we are all vaccinated.

Some people are challenging the messaging around the numbers of deaths from the pandemic; Caribbean communities believe that there is a plan afoot to lure them into taking a vaccine that could harm them. The celebrities that are pushing the positive aspects of the vaccination programme, especially from the Asian communities have an uphill task because it is not easy to undo in a year what has been perpetuated over centuries. My view is that we gently try to hear the Black and Minority Ethnic (BAME) community; they need a listening ear and a conscientious arm around them so that the virus can be defeated.

I listened to members of specific communities for example in the South Asian community pointing out that the news from the low budget delivery of communication could have been blamed for sensational headlines of the stories; usually half-truths and sharing them through other media like Facebook, WhatsApp, Twitter etc. They pointed out that there is in a constant battle with his community to convince them that vaccines are preventing hospitalisation and saving lives. A large number of the community refers to the historical abuses that people of colour were subjected to and now being asked to come to the 'rescue 'of those who oppressed them.

That is one of the arguments for mistrusting the vaccine; the counter-argument is that we are all taking the same vaccine regardless of our skin colour[22]. Incidentally, the CDCP reported from a survey conducted in the USA that 46% - 460 individuals out every 1000 Black adults said they were hesitant about being vaccinated against SARS-CoV-2 compared to 30% of white people who responded.

Responsible journalism is needed to defuse the fear that has gripped the populace around vaccinations over a long time. It is marketed by governments especially of western societies as the vehicle out of the pandemic. On the other hand, it must be noted that on its own 'the vaccine' will not eliminate the pandemic or its devastating effects; we need to follow the non-Pharmacological guidelines to complement vaccination. Responsibility; personal and corporate responsibility...

When you get a media house that reports the following as breaking news 'All UK adults will be offered first vaccine doses by September according to the foreign secretary'[23], it is irresponsible especially because the capacity to administer the vaccine is not the problem. Most accounts' problems are multi-faceted, but mainly due to the vaccines' supplies being limited and production not being fast enough. We then get the news that several elderly people in Norway died days after getting the COVID-19 vaccine... and that a faction of that number died from side effects of the vaccine, but all were nursing home patients over eighty years old - fuel for the fire of fear.

On the contrary, medical experts are to balance that by clarifying that the vaccines have minimal risk, with a tiny exclusion for the frailest, which means the professionals should consider those being vaccinated. In some countries, vaccinations are administered to very elderly and terminally ill patients, for example Norway; its health authorities are continuing to evaluate and adjust the instructions bearing the patients' prior health conditions in mind.

People who died with a terminal illness and a positive COVID-19 test had their cause of death attributed to COVID-19 even when asymptomatic, and care home deaths where no doctors

128

had visited, nor tests administered were marked as 'COVID-19' deaths.[24]

Lazy or conspiracy…

Considering this, Sky.com reports that the real figures, though hard to come by, suggest that in terms of deaths since the 1960s and contained in the Human Mortality Database (*HMD*) *between 1841 and 1960* in England and Wales (*ONS data*)[25]. Figures from Scotland being widely similar if less severe than Wales and England for all annual deaths; the only time a comparative number of deaths was recorded in England and Wales was in 1918, near the end of the first World War, which overlapped with the Spanish flu.

UK government reports that the NHS is not overwhelmed. Maybe because the measures they are taking does not speak of the high number of non-COVID-19 deaths from missed or late treatment of other conditions, the service was not coping with the weight of cases in hospitals long before the pandemic of 2020.

Then there is the jostling for position in the 'who-gets-the-vaccine-next' stakes - is it emergency workers? The [DS1] Met commissioner Cressida Dick was adamant on LBC (a radio programme) that her officers were certainly exposed. They had little or no protection from would-be spreaders of the virus. She even highlighted that several officers were coughed and spat at by members of the public claiming to have COVID –19. She had been lobbying the government on behalf of frontline officers.

Chapter 5

Cressida reassured a caller, a serving officer who postulated that some of his colleagues had fallen ill from the disease. Many officers were either sick or self-isolating, putting a strain on the service. She that she had spoken to the Home Secretary and other government members regarding the vaccination of police officers as a priority considering the various roles they were performing in the public's interest.

Many Britons' irresponsible attitude has led to reports of cyclists and other members of the public weaponising the virus, using the fear it brought to cause others to be afraid. LBC carried a clip of a male cyclist berating a motorist then spitting at her shouting derogatory slang words at her based on her ethnic background topping it off with words to the effect of "I have COVID-19." Such irresponsibility was seen in the case where a householder told the police when they attended a Hampshire property where there had been a hot tub party in progress.

Astonishingly, the occupant is reported to have told the officers they were unaware there was a pandemic going on; how unbelievable! How else could it have been to be described though; anyone saying that they did not know about the *plague* that was ravaging the entire world for the past year must be classified as irresponsible?

COVID-19 has profoundly changed our lives, causing tremendous human suffering and challenging the most basic foundations of societal well-being. Beyond the immediate impacts on health, jobs and incomes, the epidemic is increasing people's anxiety and worry, affecting their social relations, their trust in other people and in institutions, their personal security and sense of belonging.

The short and medium-term impact of COVID-19 will be particularly severe for the most disadvantaged and risk compounding existing socio-economic divides. This policy brief looks at the broad range of effects that COVID-19 will have on different aspects of people's lives, with a focus on specific population groups such as children, women and the elderly.

While governments need to act swiftly and decisively to contain the spread of the virus, countries also need to assess the impacts of the disease and the counter-measures on all aspects of people's lives, especially those most vulnerable, and integrate these distributional impacts in the response.

While racing against the clock in a complex and uncertain environment, different countries' response to the COVID-19 crisis also needs to address the well-being perspective in a holistic and integrated manner, as opposed to a sectional approach. A failure to do so risks deepening inequalities; possibly creating new divides and undermining the resilience of societies.

Chapter 6

Who is responsible?

One hundred and twenty-seven thousand deaths and counting...

Deaths in the pandemic maybe have been done to the ruling government's ten-year-old policy to be implement austerity. Cuts to essential services, including social, education, and other emergency services, have left the country unable to respond to the pandemic's demands.

'The UK government did all they could to limit the number of deaths.'[1] – Boris Johnson. It fills me with dread when the union's premier takes the podium on the day that 100,162 lives had been lost and announces that he takes full responsibility. You may ask the meaning of that statement. Has the decision making been 'flip-flop', to give it a kind spin?

To go from 18,000 hospitalisations on Christmas day to over 33,000, which is twice the number of deaths from The Blitz of World War II, as pointed out by the UK's opposition leader. Kier Starmer denounced the prime minister, accusing him of losing control after having months to prepare. He lamented, "The prime minister is not up to the job, he is just not serious, and when he encounters a problem he either wishes it away or lashes out"[2] said Kier, the leader of Her Majesty's opposition. Mr. Starmer cited leadership as a principal factor in the country having to lockdown. Canada, Brazil, and India are big economies that have seen multiple waves of the pandemic and are still gripped by it. Thousands of individuals are being infected and dying horrible deaths some having their bodies cremated in the car parks because of a lack of capacity in places like Delhi in India[3]. The fact that India makes the vast amount of the Astra Zeneca vaccine as well as manufacturing their own brand begs the question to an extent why the infection and death rate are the highest in the world.

Interestingly around Autumn 2020, the chief medical officer for England said that at the start of the pandemic there might have been about 20,000 deaths in total compared to the annual flu deaths of about 8,000[4]. He spoke about courage; he and the frontline workers would commemorate the dead when we get over this, but he cannot display any courage to own the big decisions required to lead a country in crisis.

The press Association (PA) reported on a UK-wide review that around the middle of April 2020 *'more than 3,000 deaths involving the virus occurred in a single week[5].'* With about 104,000 deaths up to January 15, 2021[6] it is difficult as there are so many issues, pain, and anguish. The absence of a comfortable atmosphere heightens the pain; hugging and gathering of the brethren at their every moment of need most times alleviates this. With March 2020 as a starting point, fast forward to April 9 2021 and the overall COVID-19 death toll in England and Wales according to the Office of National Statistics (ONS); was 137,000 – one in five of all deaths in the union during this period[7].

The rituals surrounding the marking of a death, traditions, religious or non-religious faiths must strip away so that people can manage bereavement differently. On observation of how the pandemic developed, the way people handled the death of loved ones evolved. The protocol varied from having 15 people at the church or crematorium to having a wake. A common thread is that my research has thrown up is that the celebratory tone of a loved one's life was overshadowed by the haze of death.

How we deal with death at a time like this, is a question on many lips. It has a massive effect on people when they cannot plan the funeral they would typically have wanted. It was the case that people with wishes for their passing, including carrying of coffins, having personal touches absent, so the loved ones developed grief and guilt.

It affects the mental health and well-being of those left behind while there is no recourse to counseling and care leading to a lack of empathy and closure. The lack of personal touch has led to people feeling as if they have dishonoured their loved ones…The wonders of a hug are not appreciated until we are in a position of brokenness.

Responsibility is not the British Prime Minister's strongest attribute. Early in the pandemic, he announced that the UK would roll out a 'world-beating track and trace system' to believe that for the paltry sum of £532 million. Government commissioned and built the UK Nightingale hospitals to take the NHS's pressure, using HMS soldiers with all their skills and expertise may prove why 104,000 COVID-19 deaths attributed to the UK. The ExCel Nightingale hospital was the COVID-19 field hospital to be erected in only nine days and opened with grandeur by the heir to the throne in England; Prince Charles, NHS experts and soldiers, made it possible.

Unfortunately, given the requirement for these facilities, staffed by specialists to man ventilators, the "elated" nurses housed in nearby hotels were brushing up their knowledge by e-learning platforms. Patient numbers were rising very rapidly in April 2020 and that increased the need for more of these facilities to the set up in other areas around the UK.

The panic-induced decision was observed as a costly mistake because the Nightingale hospital in Manchester treated 100 patients in 2020, while Nightingale Exeter treated 29 patients during the peak month when the UK topped the 100,000 COVID-19 deaths. It was later earmarked to be used as a centre for diagnostics and could be converted to assist the surrounding hospitals deal with backlogs in routine hospital care. In the ExCel Centre 4000 capacity facility, the Sunderland and Birmingham treated no patients whatsoever; Bristol and Harrogate used as receptacles for other patients and services.

Parliamentarians will need to scrutinise these white elephants, but in the context of where the country's hospitals are gripped intensely by the pressure on staff. Also, the astronomic level of demand on the treatment and alarming transmission rate, it will be some time away. Lessons from this pandemic must be learned and quickly; it is already apparent that some people who oversee the health service failed miserably to get their heads around how crucial people who work in the National Health Service are in society (NHS).

Nurses and other health care staff are struggling to cope financially; this was the case before the pandemic that has escalated during it. Band five nurses coming out of University with a student loan and all other living costs simply do not have the resources to feed themselves, much less afford to rent or worse yet buy a house. Mike Adams, Royal College of Nursing [RCN] Director for England, working hard in the interest of nurses. All this while being aware of the challenges and pressures that many nurses face in their day-to-day lives called on government to be mindful.

As we unmask corona, we continue to see the need to keep up building the RCN community to help develop both working lives and patient care. The governments of countries should begin to believe in a strong health system where kindness and understanding can be employed in any situation and where nursing staff and other health care staff should always try to show this in how they interact and care for patients, service users, and each other in whatever part of the world they find themselves.

The absence of skilled labour explains why the Nightingale hospital at ExCel London was destined to hit a brick wall [fail]. The professionals, doctors and nurses who work in intensive care units [ICUs] are very experienced with several years working as individuals and working in teams. They are not easy to toss together [assemble] because of cultures and methods that get on with the job of caring. The feat to get 4000 specialist beds into a facility in the East End of London, regardless of how good it appeared at the time, was going to be hard - having established that, it is safe to say that it would never have been feasible for the military theme hospital to adequately provide the service that a purpose-built established hospital would give.

The UK prime minister had his life saved from the Corona virus in the 'world-beating' Guys and St Thomas' Hospital. He made a point of acknowledging the nurses from ethnic backgrounds who staged vigils around his bed. The Nightingales were just fantastic; I say this because the nurses and other staff necessary to make them work were not available from other overextended hospitals. Supply was way below demand, and the economics of that are clear; it leads to shortages and inefficiencies in this case.

Kate Bingham appointed as chairperson of the UK Vaccine Taskforce that was set up and manage the path towards vaccine roll out in the UK remained demonised when things were toxic in the last quarter of 2020[8]. However, because she is married to the Treasury minister named Jesse Norman, the daggers came out when the cracks appeared in the government's handling of the pandemic. Her appointment was vindicated in a big way as UK was among the first in the world to roll out large scale vaccination programmes at the end of 2020.

It was a paradox because, whilst all this unfolded, Ms. Bingham was able to show backers details about vaccines her team was monitoring and by the first quarter of 2021 the UK was leading Europe and only behind Israel in the vaccinating of their population. This was so because government messaging has done a fantastic job with vaccines' procurement by most accounts. It appears the UK is getting on with the business of managing, and the vaccine rollout is the flicker of light that is visible as we meander through this dark tunnel named corona virus pandemic.

She was later hailed as a champion when the chaos unfolded from the onset of winter 2020 with the countries of the EU left behind in the acquisition of the vaccines for their populations. I guess Kate Bingham will become Baroness Bingham before long…

Under the cover of COVID-19, the Amazon is attacked…:

The Amazon rainforest is under attack masked by the veil of COVID-19. Deforestation is at its highest rate for at least 10 years, during which time (up until a year ago) the loggers and prospectors were only able to operate under the cover of darkness brought about by the pandemic. Environmental fines of hundreds of thousands of pounds for deforestation offences of businesspeople, former and current mayors show the scope of the problem. The new regime headed by president Bolsonaro offer protection for these deforesters by rewriting the laws set up to protect the trees and animals and talked about opening the forest for development. The only known tribe that has never had contact with civilisation has been under serious pressure as a result.

In 2012 the Brazilian government managed to implement laws that reduced and brought deforestation under control and the benefit to both plant and animal welfare was immense. Patrols and government bulldozers cleared away the loggers who were depleting the forest. It showed the government could affect the state the world's 'lungs'; a name I coin for the Amazon since its trees provided so much of the oxygen whilst removing the carbon dioxide from the air. Over time, records show that nearly half a million square kilometers of forest have been razed in about 35yrs...

Politics played its slight hand when the ruling government in one of the most densely populated countries in South America was filmed in a meeting plotting to use the COVID-19 mask to cover the removal of many of the protections that were in place.

The media had a field day with the information, but the ruling party claimed the decision was to simplify the existing rules, but the reality was that after the cabinet meeting in which ministers schemed to remove all the protections – they managed to remove the protections from a lot of the forested areas in the country. It has turned out that the forest has returned to the times where the support for the patrols was low. Gold prospectors and gold mines returned to mainstream and no longer felt scared of persecution because they felt the president would protect them. This led to lawlessness and riots between loggers, prospectors and forest environmental patrol officers came under attack while the police (who are loyal to the president) stood by and watched.

Professor Simon Wang, reader of Climate dynamics and prediction, University of Utah, confirmed the trend for the past

20 yrs. His work has shown that the climate is in a constant
state of change under the influence of biological and physical
forces. Heat waves kicks off the wildfires in North America
and other continents; these trends have shown no signs of
stopping. The forests have been stopped from burning and
controlling itself. This is because of inhabitation...

Arizona – fire fighters die when fighting fires in California – a
dangerous place to live (high profile people pay a lot to live
there). Large parts are desolate with much potential to burn; a
direct impact of Climate change – reality –warming outside of
'mother nature's control'; records temperatures, precipitation –
low pressure system. The European floods and fires have been
unprecedented, never before seen at these levels.. Failure to
invest in Green energy, we must spend in order to avert
disasters like floods and heat waves currently experienced.

Managing Grief

The dictionary defines grief as a noun meaning 'intense sorrow,
especially caused by someone's death'[1]— Lianna Champ. The
funeral director defines it is the normal and natural reaction we
experience when we lose someone or something we value;
when we lose our familiar patterns of behaviour, we grieve
results.

When losing someone significant, the funeral is the opportunity to celebrate a person's whole life that we have lost. People use it to express their love and devotion to their family member.

We must celebrate life, not just wait until death; people live over an extended period, and people must embrace that time with loved ones. Sound advice is that we should not allow COVID-19 to hijack our loved ones; the shared and happy experiences must be the fuel that keeps the flame of love for our family going. In life, as in death, we expect to do what is right for our loved ones.

The lack of personal touch is massive, and the funeral directors are crucial in helping people through these times. Funerals are conducted virtually, and the undertakers have the most contact with the deceased even when the closest family is not allowed.

So, they need to be trained and skilled to console and work with grieving families; there must be a profession's passion; it is vocational. Grief is personal, requires understanding, and the director must support those grieving. They must guide families through it so that they can come through the other end and emerge stronger, wiser, and kinder to the people in their lives.

There is no guarantee that the people we have in our lives today, will be around tomorrow. The five stages of grief (Elisabeth Kübler-Ross) are denial, anger, bargaining, depression, and acceptance[2]. These help to explain (but not justify) why in my grieving I may become angry with God, enraged by the apparent unfairness of his will. Why did he take my loved one?

At certain other stages, I may seek to bargain with God, I repent of the wrong things I did, trying to be a better version of myself. I fast and pray making all kinds of promises in the process, trying to convince God he should change His mind. One writer refers to this as 'bribery of the infinite'. After offloading my anger on the creator and failing to bribe Him, there are only two choices left for me: depression or acceptance.

Where would I be better?

Do I want to be, wallowing in self-pity, blaming others, taking offense, which is usually selfish, and giving up the desire to fight?

Do I want God to change His Word, to appease me? Is depression an option?

We want God to do something for us besides the Finished Work of Christ. One writer states that 'We have all spent time in self-pity, and when we go there the demons love it. They know it is one of the most dangerous places a Christian can go, because if we stay there, we will end up blaming God'[1]

Or instead of the 'Poor old me, I have been fighting this feeling forever', we pray for God to help us to be gentle on ourselves as we mourn our loss. It would be a joy to ask for help to grieve well, for our desires to be able to coexist with His desires, my will with His will, and my acceptance with the goodness of God's sovereign purposes.

Bereavement gifts play a big part in the process, and I will list several options available provided by Champ funeral services' CEO, Lianna Champ[2]:

1. Flowers

There are more requests for donations than flowers, so those that decorate the casket are mainly from family. A floral arrangement sent to the family home is a thoughtful way to show you care, and flowers can brighten their surroundings.

2. Food

When we are bereaved, it can be challenging to cope with the most basic of tasks. Cooking takes a back seat as we can get pulled in so many different directions. A timely casserole or lovely home-baked cake to share with visitors is usually appreciated.

3. Donate Your Time

Helping with shopping and ironing and general chores is invaluable. Set a time to do this and keep to it. Gifts of time are lovely and always welcome.

4. Memory Candle

A candle makes a beautiful bereavement gift, and the candle can be a light on remembrance days as well as those times when we connect and harness our thoughts in the most spiritual of ways. The flame signifies the eternal nature of spirit even beyond life.

5. Picture Frame

Preserving a beautiful photo is a lovely gesture and can evoke memories of happy times.

6. Memory Box or Jar

An on-going, unfolding gift where favourite memories written down is recalled on decorated pieces of paper and placed in a memory box. Selected items can also follow — a lock of hair, photo, pebbles, crystal heart or anything that has meaning for you. It is lovely to open the memory box on those occasions when you need to feel close to the person you have lost.

7. Plant or Shrub

Another lovely bereavement gift can be presented in a beautiful tub or planted in the garden, especially for the outdoors and garden lovers. If cremation has been the choice, the ashes or a portion can be mixed in with the soil 'immortalising' the loved one.

8. Tree Bauble

This personalised bauble with a loving message on it can be hung indoors or outdoors all year round. Some trinkets can be personalised for Christmas to hang on a Christmas tree. Christmas is family time and hanging a personalised bauble can help bring us into communion with those we have lost. We will have a constant reminder every time we see the bauble.

9. Memory Teddy Bear

Our love for someone we lose is stored internally, and it does not always have somewhere to go. A bear is lovely as we can hug it and be honest; everyone loves a bear. Buy or make a top or baby for the bear and have the deceased person's name onto the top in embroidery Bears signifies cuddle and a much-needed hug, especially if we need a good cry.

10. Wildflower Tokens

A symbol of life continues. Planting something is incredibly special. It casts our thoughts to our loved one while giving energy to their spirit. Watching the flowers grow also evokes our love for the person[3].

11. Memorial Garden Ornament

This is a special bereavement gift for nature lovers, the outdoors, or their garden. A memorial sundial or a bird table makes a lovely gift that can allow for enjoyment for many years. They can help connect us with the rhythms of nature, reminding us of the beauty of life and the sun's warmth.

12. Cushion

A cushion could be an item made from cuts of favourite pieces of clothing of the person who has died. Cushions can create a unique, personal bereavement gift.

Chapter 6

13. Jewellery

There are many beautiful jewellery bereavement gifts available, from fingerprint items to lockets and hearts for photographs, locks of hair and grains/ashes of cremated remains - a beautiful way to remember and a lovely keepsake.

14. Spa Treatment Gift Voucher

When someone is grieving, there is nothing more comforting than the feeling of being wrapped in cotton wool. A gift voucher for a soothing massage or healing therapy can be most welcome.

15. Crystals

Crystals are a beautiful bereavement gift and are chosen for a particular area of focus e.g., rose quartz is for healing and love, and can be handheld for moments of reflection, meditation, and spirituality.

With people from many sectors of society crying out for the opportunity to bury their lost loved ones and say their goodbyes properly. Governments in countries from Jamaica to the United Kingdom have tip toed around the issue and people are not able to grieve. It has gone on for so long that the families and friends of these people are now at the point where the will to follow protocol has been strained to breaking point.

COVID-19 has unmasked a deluge of underlying illnesses affecting people in these societies. Patients are saddled with comorbidities (simultaneous presence of two or more diseases or medical conditions).Caribbean people appear to be seriously impacted by the presence of Diabetes Mellitus (type 2) in the region.

In the British Isles there was a discussion about increasing the numbers of mourners from thirty to making it dependent on the capacity of the venues a month earlier than originally planned. This might be down to the relative success of the vaccination programme in these isles[4].

An example of the concern was a woman who reported that her friend went to a party at Christmas time and got infected; she knew it was not right. This woman, who I will call Dawn, a teacher, said her friend, who I will call Delores, took the virus home from the party to her elderly parents, John and Jill; they were shielding.

She infected them because she interacted with people with the virus, but the symptoms appeared mild. The people from the party Delores attended had all tested positive. I found it heartening to hear Dawn report how every person that participated in the party got infected, and her friend went for a test and found that she might have been responsible for her parents, who had been married for 60 years, contracting the virus. The father got out of the hospital and must now live with his mental trauma: his wife leaving the house in an ambulance, going to hospital, dying, and buried without him ever seeing her again.

Society's responsibility for the people has never been greater; the scenario I just mentioned is played out in communities worldwide, especially in the western world in this pandemic.

Chapter 6

Many people do not take their role as citizens seriously; it can be almost referred to as chronic selfishness syndrome, to coin a phrase. Doctor Ben White, who was helping a radio station with the truth about the pandemic from the 'shop floor/battlefield/warzone', spoke to a journalist.

I opined that he felt that my scenario above resulted from social media reneging on its responsibility to police and shut-down content that promotes a lack of adherence to the rules that will keep us all safe. The pain felt by this acute doctor was implicated in the fight for young doctors' rights who have nothing but duty in carrying out the role as a doctor in a pandemic.

He is adamant that people who cause the mayhem need to be brought to book while being reminded that the situation prevents this from happening because of the laws of the land. Doctors and nurses are the last line of defence that we have as a nation, and they are at breaking point because every human being's responsibility is to preserve self and be mindful of their fellow man...

'Let each of you look not only to his interests but also to the interests of others.'[5]

.... We should probably look to these quotations on wisdom; evidence is also available in both the Jewish Torah and the Muslim Quran. It is a maxim all of us should never forget.

'He who saves a single life saves the world entire.'[6]

Afterword

This book opened explaining the mission; to set some things straight in the time of the biggest pandemic in the last hundred years. I passionately believe that the pandemic that allegedly had its Genesis in Wuhan, China impacted and continue to impact the entire world in more ways than meet the eye. Amongst other things like, the USA's election, and the United Kingdom's exit from the European Union (EU), the European Football Cup completion and the Olympic Games were all due to be happening at the same time. The idea that the SARS-COV- 2 was synthesised (made in a lab) has not gone away, with high profile diplomats reserving that opinion even late in 2021.

Prominent scientists put their signatures to a published journal article calling into question the transparency of the investigations into the origins of the virus that caused COVID-19. It means that the Wuhan lab leak theory of which I spoke has again gained momentum worldwide with support from public officials and academics. The Biden administration has called from the intelligence officials in America to 'redouble' efforts to uncover the truth...

God's Word tells us that '*greater is He who is in us than he is in the world*' (see 1 John 4:4). God has a plan for America and the world for this season. It is not all about electing a new president, but shifting things in America and the world at large where there is obviously serious trouble. God has been forgotten or deliberately removed. The human conscience failing, deprived of its godly element, has been the factor shaping all major crimes and debauchery in our society – 'People have forgotten God'...

Did we see the reawakening of white evangelicalism during the last four years in the USA? White Christian America stood by its man – Donald Trump. They were the ticket on which he was elected and they failed to get him re-elected, but not without a fight. The 'born again' found it in their heart to tolerate the man who just couldn't do any wrong by them. Trump walking out and about without a mask in the White House's grounds after he was hospitalised at the height of a pandemic, is a stark reminder. He showed a total lack of regard for those around him when he returned to the White House, recklessly declaring that there is nothing to fear from COVID-19.

People died from the coronavirus at the time of the election in America, the total deaths numbering around a quarter of a million. The commander in chief (Trump) hindered medical practitioners trying to save lives by spouting misinformation to the public, yet he could do no wrong in the eyes of the Evangelicals.

Did Nostradamus predict what we are seeing unfold as far back as 1555? Or other claimants from the likes of novelist Dean Koontz who predicted the epidemic in his 1981 book entitled *'Eyes of Darkness'*? Or is it the blind mystic known as Baba Vanga christened Vangeliya Pandeva Gushterova in Bulgaria? On October 3, a raft of her followers considers 1911 to be equal to Nostradamus. She is credited with predicting the

Russian submarine Kursk and online sources' sinking, saying that she predicted the deadly corona (SARS-CoV2) virus before she died in 1996.

Even though there are no documents to verify her opinions, she is supposed to have announced that the Russian state would produce leaders who would change the world. She even said there would be a cure found for cancer early in the 21st century - "the day will come, and cancer will be chained in iron chains". She is supposed to have declared also that *'the medicine against cancer should contain much iron'*...

The novel SARS-CoV-2 appeared seemingly out of nowhere in 2019, rapidly infecting thousands of people in the capital of Hubei province, Wuhan City. Despite the Chinese's government's attempts to stop the virus from spreading beyond the country's borders, infections soon flared in other parts of Asia, Europe, Africa, and the Americas. By January 4, the virus had infected more than 85.2 million people and even made its way to a remote research station in Antarctica, meaning COVID-19 had officially spread to every corner of the globe.

Despite the best efforts, more than 1.94 million people globally have died, and new strains of the virus appeared in the UK at the time of writing with the Delta variant (first attributed to India) wreaking havoc worldwide.

The race between the virus and the vaccine has intensified with developing countries lacking behind. It should be the injection versus the infection with a view to getting the world back to a place where thing could return to some amount of normalcy. There is tension between countries; Canada, the EU led by France, Germany and a few big economies that have suspended the rollout of the Astra Zeneca (AZ) vaccine.

There are people hesitating and others procrastinating because they have a preferred vaccine; the way pandemics work, it would be foolish to refuse the offer of a vaccine, regardless of the producer. The best vaccine is the one that is available, a prominent member of the society opined that *'no one is safe until everyone is safe'* a sentiment I wholeheartedly share.

The figures from studies in the Guardian newspaper show that 9 of 10 people in countries like the United Kingdom continue to wear masks. In England, the parliamentarians ditched masks in enclosed spaces at the recall of parliament over the Afghanistan debacle the lack of leadership presented itself. There are dissenting voices in my immediate environment echoing the anti-mask rhetoric banking on the luxury of youth. Contrast that with the approach in Wales where a greater sector of the population continues to wear masks as they ease out of their latest lockdown.

Numbers of infections and hospitalisations reflect the level of responsibility on display by different societies. The messaging continues to be mixed and that has led to many, many people in a great number of western societies not bothering to wear the mask…

Professional footballers in the UK and NFL players in the states are displaying resistance to vaccination. It might be down to the fact that their jobs mandate that they are in the highest level of fitness. They could be forgiven for saying that they do not have enough long term evidence on the long term effects of the COVID-19 vaccination.

On the other hand, with 2019 figures showing that around 70% of NFL players are black and the premiership doubling the number of BAME players from 16.5% over the last 20 years or so. The demographics of the people that have been affected most severely over the period of the ongoing pandemic show this section of the society bore the blunt of the suffering.

Is it any wonder that these fit athletes are taking an avant-garde view in a time where uncertainties and indiscretion abound? It reflects the narrative forwarded by the 25 – 35 age groups that are most hesitant to vaccination. Authorities reported that numerous sources continue to monitor the situation but encounter the daily dilemma in which the fight against misinformation, historical truths about abuse on communities perpetrated by governmental agencies.

An effort to defog society's need for shared responsibly is best seen in the fact that the sports world is a microcosm of our larger society. Elite athletes usually are the front facing representatives of the charter or league, and support or uncertainty can change the minds of a significant number of fans in many instances idolise them. In a time when public attitude in the world has improved, it could be turbo charged if the messaging from leaders of all persuasions flew the flag for: vaccination, mask wearing and other precautionary measures as essential elements in the fight against the pandemic...

Afterword

Think about societies across the world where the people have modest ways of making ends meet. Your typical street vendor, soup seller or fruit juice peddler that make their living from setting up where there is a constant footfall. People with children to feed and utility bills to pay, having no other source of income when restrictions brought about by the global pandemic cripple their existence.

Many understand the efforts being made are designed to increase the fight against the invisible enemy besieging the globe. There is a confusion in the minds of individuals is why there seems to be different rules for different folks...policies lacking consistency. Take the case of Prince Charles of England, who has been reported saying he will wear a mask if he is asked to in the height of a global pandemic.

We could look at the Jamaican government allowing tourists to flock the island and party while the locals are given non-movement orders and schools unable to resume face-to-face lessons. Countries of the world have a traffic light system that allows movement across borders. USA citizens are allowed into the United Kingdom but the citizens of the UK are prevented from making the trip the other way. There are still travel restrictions in place for me travelling from the United Kingdom to United States and I am told by the travel industry that United States travelers are still allowed to enter Britain. How is this allowed to happen? One rule for some, another rule for others...

Researchers from Kings College London have backed up the findings released by the Lancet, stating that two doses of the vaccines just about halved the chance of adults being affected by long term effects of 'coronavirus' [Long COVID -19]. This data reiterated the point that the risk hospitalisation was likely to be up to 73% less and all chances of severe COVID-19 symptoms saw reductions of nearly 33%[2].

The lead investigator of the ZOE COVID study; Professor Tim Spector, stated that *'We are encouraging people to get their second vaccine as soon as they can'*[3]. This encouragement goes for those who are hesitant and are yet to be vaccinated. He followed up with this assurance. 'Vaccinations are rapidly reducing the chances of people getting Long Covid …'[4]

Regular citizens for the most part would never ask their government for handouts, but instead aspire to go out and get their own metaphorical bread. These people have been made to take part in a global experiment to prop up the economies of the world; the general populations are suffering as a result…

When one of the world's finest Formula One racing drivers can make the news headlines for something outside of racing we take notice. 'Big Pharma' companies are incensed because he (Sir Lewis Hamilton) has released his new CBD line of products. 'How dare this little black boy from Stevenage?' Big Pharma may be thinking. The pharmaceutical giants are threatening lawsuits against Lewis Hamilton and his partners, claiming they violated their contracts and are undercutting their prices. Interesting!

The racing great has said that after receiving much from the sport; it is fitting that he should give something back and

Afterword

thought the *Green CBD Gummy Bears* (GCGB) project was the ideal way. His transgression is the effort to make to make life as pain-free for as many people as possible. The records show that the product has been flying off the shelves and thousands are being helped…sounds like shared responsibility to me.

Glaxo Smith Kliene and Pfizer are most angry after their sales decreased remarkably and are calling for Sir Lewis and his GCGB partners to be brought to justice. Their crime was making treatment available over the counter that could help the masses suffering from chronic pain. The Mail Online reported that the big companies stated: 'we are happy Mr. Hamilton found something to replace prescriptions, but his announcement was a direct breach of contract.' The next part of the statement will blow you away; the report continued, saying his sponsors should drop him immediately and he should formally apologise.[1]

Sir Lewis, in his usual steely style retorted that Green CBD Gummy Bears has helped him and his family succeed and cope with ailments so he had immense confidence making it available to everyone. Incidentally, the word was that his wellness line is up to 86% less expensive and up to four times more effective than other brands. Also, in a television appearance, he offered free bags to viewers defending the product and reiterated that he will not be intimidated…Shared responsibility 101.

Collective consciousness is required as a consequence of the veil being yanked from the faces of a huge sector of our society…

In short, the world in which we currently live in is a bit of a shambles, and the book which you have just gone through has hopefully shown that. Now armed with this knowledge, you should be able to confidently participate in coronavirus-based conversations.

About the author

Derrick H. Shortridge is an experienced educator, science teacher; counselor and Christian young people advocate who lives in the UK. However, he travels back and forth to his native Jamaica and Florida (where much of his family live) regularly.

He has been an educator for all his working life and over the past six years has committed his life and work to helping the world through Christian pursuits. He claims to still get a buzz when "the light bulb" moments arrive and they very often do.

As a secondary school science teacher and a force not to be reckoned with, his reputation went before him in the school as a teacher not to mess about with, whether you were a student in his class or a student making noise in his corridor.

However, this reputation was earned based on students having the utmost respect for his time, teaching acumen and genuine father-like authority. If you happen to get a sharp reprimand by Derrick Shortridge, you knew you would be impacted for life.

He has captured episodes traversing education and societal discussions on not just the science of coronavirus but also the implications of the pandemic. In his first publication, a unique book in popular science that does not shy away from drawing parallels between biblical references and the current situation we are in.

Derrick offers the opportunity for a crash course in virology without ever having to attend a formal virology course or seminar. He captures how COVID-19 has impacted the globe in a major way and what it tells us about the brokenness of society as we know it.

He is driven by the logic of Dr. Frances Cress Welsing who said "we're the only people on this planet who have been taught to sing and praise our demeanment. 'I'm a bitch, I'm a hoe, I'm a gangster, a thug, and I'm a dog.' If you can train people to demean and degrade themselves, you can oppress them forever. You can even programme them to kill themselves and they won't even understand what happened."

Derrick is a family man, father to two sons and a daughter. He transformed his life turning the difficult early experiences he into positive life lessons.

Notes

Prologue

1. LBC – Leading Britain's conversation
2. Dr. David Jeremiah, *"Is this the end*?" 2018;
3. Ibid
4. NKJV
5. Ecclesiastes 8:15 – bible hub.com
6. John 10:10 - NKJV
7. Rom 12:12 - NKJV
8. Col: 4-5
9. 2 Cor 3:12
10. 2 Thessalonians 1:3
11. 2 Thessalonians 2:16-17
12. *Jeremiah 29:11; The NKJV*
13. *Ibid*
14. https://swissmodel.expasy.org/repository/species/2697049.
15. https://blast.ncbi.nlm.nih.gov/Blast.cgi.
16. Global Health News Wire, "The covid-19 coronavirus epidemic has a natural origin, scientists say," *https://globalhealthnewswire.com/*

Chapter one

Education for basic understanding

1. Elana Pearl Ben-Joseph.MD, "What Are the Types of Germs," March 2020;

https://kidshealth.org/en/parents/germs.html

2. Reviewed by Cameron White, M.D.mph, "Am I Too Sick or Contagious to Work?" May2019;

https://www.healthline.com/health/cold-flu/contagious#when-to-stay-home.

3. "Virology," September 2021;

https://www.nature.com/subjectsvirology

4. Dr. Joe Francis, "COVID-19, Coronavirus, and Creation Virology," March 2020,

https://answersingenesis.org/coronavirus/covid19-coronavirus-and-creation-virology//#fn_1

5. Ibid

6. Swiss model repository;

https://swissmodel.expasy.org/repository/species/26
97049

Notes

How does severe acute respiratory syndrome SARS – CoV-2 cause disease?

1.   The Guardian, 'Hands. Face. Space': UK government to relaunch Covid-19 slogan; September 2020; https://www.theguardian.com/world/2020/sep/09/hands-face-space-uk-government-to-relaunch-covid-19-slogan

2.   UK Research and Innovation, "What is coronavirus? The different types of corona viruses," March 2020, https://coronavirusexplained.ukri.org/en/article/cad0003/

3.   "The species Severe acute respiratory syndrome-related coronavirus: classifying 2019-nCoV and naming it SARS-CoV-2", March 2020, https://www.nature.com/articles/s41564-020-0695-z

4.   Esther Landhuris, "An Immune Protein could prevent COVID-19 - if it's given at the right time," September 2020; https://www.scientificamerican.com/article/an-immune-protein-could-prevent-severe-covid-19-if-it-is-given-at-the-right-time1/

5.   "COVID-19 research: a year of scientific milestones," May 2021, https://www.nature.com/articles/d41586-020-00502-w

6.   Krishna Sriram, Paul Insel, Rohit Loomba, "What is the ACE2 receptor, how is it connected to coronavirus and what

might it be key to treating COVID-19? The expert explained."
May 2020,
https://theconversation.com/what-is-the-ace2-receptor-how-is-it-connected-to-coronavirus-and-why-might-it-be-key-to-treating-covid-19-the-experts-explain-136928

7.   WHO, "How is COVID-19 transmitted?" July 2020,
https://www.who.int/vietnam/news/detail/14-07-2020-q-a-how-is-covid-19-transmitted

Vaccine Efficacy explained

1. Ewen Callaway, "Coronavirus variants get Greek names-but will scientists use them?" June 2021,
    https://www.nature.com/articles/d41586-021-01483-0

2. Ibid

3. Ibid

4. CNN Health, "Detroit vaccines: Mayor declines Johnson & Johnson," March2021,
    https://edition.cnn.com/2021/03/04/health/detroit-mayor-johnson-and-johnson-vaccine/index.html

5. John Miller, "Shot in the dark: Early COVID-19 vaccine efficacy explained," November2020,
    https://www.reuters.com/article/us-health-coronavirus-vaccine-efficacy-e-idUSKBN27S2EI

6. Mary Ramsay, "COVID-19: analysing first vaccine effectiveness in the UK," February2021, https://publichealthmatters.blog.gov.uk/2021/02/23/covid-19-analysing-first-vaccine-effectiveness-in-the-uk/

What happens in a pandemic...

1.   1 Peter 1:6-8
www.Biblehub.com

2.   "Why soap works –The New York Times," March 2020.
https://www.nytimes.com/2020/03/13/health/soap-coronavirus-handwashing-germs.html

3.   WHO, "Vector – borne diseases," March 2020.
https://www.who.int/news-room/fact-sheets/detail/vector-borne-diseases

4.   "SARS-CoV-2 jumping the species barrier: Zoonotic lessons from SARS, MERS and recent advances to combat the pandemic virus," September-October 2020,
https://www.ncbi.nlm.nih.gov/pmc/articles/PMC7396141/

5.   Smriti Mallapaty, "Meet the scientists investigating the origins of the COVID-19 pandemic," December 2020,
https://www.nature.com/articles/d41586-020-03402-1

6.   Ibid

7.   WHO Director-General's opening remarks at the media briefing on COVID-19, March 2020, https://www.who.int/director-general/speeches/detail/who-director-general-s-opening-remarks-at-the-media-briefing-on-covid-19---3-march-2020

8.   David JP Phillips, TEDx Stockholm, "The magical science of storytelling," March 2017, https://www.youtube.com/watch?v=Nj-hdQMa3uA

9.   Saad Shakir; "How pharmocovigilance need to adapt in order to handle the challenges of advanced therapies and the COVID-19 pandemic," https://www.dsru.org/how-pharmacovigilance-needs-to-adapt-in-order-to-handle-the-challenges-of-advanced-therapies-and-the-covid-19-pandemic/

10.   Jeanne P. Spencer, MD. Ruth H. Trondsen Ppawlowski, MD. And Stephanie Thomas, PharmD, Conemaugh Family Medicine Residency program, Johnstown, Pennsylvania; "Vaccine Adverse Events: Separating Myth form Reality," June 2017, https://www.aafp.org/afp/2017/0615/p786.html

11.   Immunochromography Guide – Creative Diagnostics, https://www.creative-diagnostics.com/Immunochromatography-guide.htm

12.   Emma B. Hodcroft, PhD; Adam S. Lauring, MD, PhD; COVID-19 Resource Center, "Genetic variants of SARS-CoV-2 – What do they mean?" Jan 2021; https://jamanetwork.com/journals/jama/fullarticle/2775006

13.   Types of Influenza, Center for Disease Control and Prevention (CDC), https://www.cdc.gov/flu/about/viruses/types.htm

14.   Published online, "Influenza A Virus Cell Entry, Replication, virion assembly and movement," July 2018, https://www.ncbi.nlm.nih.gov/pmc/articles/PMC6062596/

15.   Liverpool University, "Liverpool Responds: Research, Action!" July 2020, https://www.facebook.com/watch/live/?v=570942983605176&ref=watch_permalink

Be Educated ...Get vaccinated

1. WHO, "How vaccines work?" December 2020, https://www.who.int/news-room/feature-stories/detail/how-do-vaccines-work

2. Greig Watson, BBC News; "The anti-vaccination movement that gripped Victorian England," December 2019; https://www.bbc.co.uk/news/uk-england-leicestershire-50713991

3. Stefan Riedel; MD, PhD; cited in other articles in PMC; "Edward Jenner and the history of smallpox and vaccination,"
https://www.ncbi.nlm.nih.gov/pmc/articles/PMC12006964

4.   CDC, "Reconstruction of the1918 Influenza Pandemic Virus,"
https://www.cdc.gov/flu/about/qa/1918flupandemic.htm

5.   (See note 3)

6.   Christopher Charlton, "The Leicester demonstration of 1885-Local Population,"
http://www.localpopulationstudies.org.uk/PDF/LPS30/LPS30_1983_60-66.pdf

7.   Royal Cornwall gazette, December 1886

8.   Laurrie Clarke, "Would a mandatory COVID-19 vaccine be ethically justified?" December 2020,
https://www.newstatesman.com/science-tech/coronavirus/2020/12/would-mandatory-covid-19-vaccine-be-ethically-justified

9. Hosea 4:5-7, NKJV

Notes

Vaccinations are wonderful...

1.   Dr. Martin Boatman et al. "How does the human body fight a viral infection?" September 2020, *https://www.open.edu/openlearn/science-maths-technology/biology/how-does-the-human-body-fight-viral-infection*

2.   Greig Watson, BBC News, "The anti-vaccination movement that gripped Victorian England," December 2019; https://www.bbc.co.uk/news/uk-england-leicestershire-50713991

3.   Conspiracy Theorist Piers Corbyn tells a crowd of unmasked protesters, "Covid is a hoax," The Sun, November 2020 https://www.thesun.co.uk/news/uknews/13946769/piers-corbyn-arrested-covid-conspiracy-pamphlet-vaccinations/

https://www.thesun.co.uk/news/uknews/13946769/piers-corbyn-arrested-covid-conspiracy-pamphlet-vaccinations/

4. Johns Hopkins, Bloomberg School of Public Health, Gypsyamber D'Souza, David Dowdy; "What is Herd Immunity and How Can We Achieve It With COVID-19?" April 2021, *https://publichealth.jhu.edu/2021/what-is-heard-immunity-and-how-can-we-achieve-it-with-covid-19*

5. Christine Aschwanden; "Five reasons why COVID herd immunity is probably impossible," March 2021, https://www.nature.com/articles/d41586-021-00728-2

Artificially Acquired Passive Immunity

1. "War on COVID with Dr. Ramon Arscott," June 2021, https://www.youtube.com/watch?v=dqfZ_tIqCuA

2. "Active vs. Passive Immunity: Differences and Definition," May 2020, Images for a diagram showing a type of active immunity... https://www.technologynetworks.com/immunology/articles/active-vs-passive-immunity-differences-and-definition-335112

3. Ibid

What is active immunity?

1. 'Active vs. Passive Immunity: Differences and Definition', May 2020, Images for a diagram showing a type of active immunity... *https://www.technologynetworks.com/immunology/articles/active-vs-passive-immunity-differences-and-definition-335112*

2. Ibid

Notes

Vaccine Storage/shortage

1.   Selena Simmons-Duffin, "Why Does Pfizer's COVID-19 needs to be colder than Antartica?" November 2020, *https://www.npr.org/sections/health-shots/2020/11/17/935563377/why-does-pfizers-covid-19-vaccine-need-to-be-kept-colder-than-antarctica?t=1631261330969*

2.   Caroline Brogan, "Q&A: Cold chains, COVID-19 vaccine and reaching low-income countries," December 2020, Imperial College London; *https://www.imperial.ac.uk/news/209993/qa-cold-chains-covid-19-vaccines-reaching/*

3.   "Pfizer and Bio N Tech conclude phase 3 study of COVID-19 vaccine candidate, meeting and all primary efficacy endpoints," November 2020, *https://www.pfizer.com/news/press-release/press-release-detail/pfizer-and-biontech-conclude-phase-3-study-covid-19-vaccine*

4.   The Wall Street journal, "Supply – chain obstacles led to last month's cut to Pfizer's COVD-19 Vaccine – Rollout targets, Costas Paris," December 2020; *https://www.wsj.com/articles/pfizer-slashed-its-covid-19-vaccine-rollout-target-after-facing-supply-chain-obstacles-11607027787*

5.   'Packing vaccines for transport in emergencies', *https://www.cdc.gov/vaccines/recs/storage/downloads/emergency-transport.pdf*

6.   "Johnson & Johnson Announces Data to support boosting its single-shot COVID-19 vaccine," March 2021, *https://www.jnj.com/johnson-johnson-covid-19-vaccine-authorized-by-u-s-fda-for-emergency-usefirst-single-shot-vaccine-in-fight-against-global-pandemic*

7.   Andrew J. Pollard & Else M. Biker, Nature reviews immunology; "A guide to vaccinology: from basic principles to new developments," *https://www.nature.com/articles/s41577-020-00479-7*

8.   Yuan-Chuan Chen, Hwei-Fang Cheng, Yi-Chen Yang and Ming-Kung Yuh, "Biotechnologies Applied in Biomedical Vaccines," November 2016; *https://www.intechopen.com/chapters/55860*

9.   "AstraZeneca vaccine document shows a limit to no-profit pledge", The Financial Times, July 2021, *https://www.ft.com/content/d9eb2e1f-965f-462c-bfcd-ca4339. Confirmed cases of COVID-19cb5ca9*

10.   Public Health England (PHE), "Confirmed cases of COVID-19 variants indentified in UK," Published December 2020, Last updated September 2021; *https://www.gov.uk/government/news/confirmed-cases-of-covid-19-variants-identified-in-uk*

Chapter Two

Notes

To mask or not to mask...

1.   Science, Tech & Health/Biology & Genetics "A viral 'family tree'," – Published on September 01, 2016; https://www.bc.edu/bc-web/bcnews/science-tech-and-health/biology-and-genetics/tracking-ancient-viruses1.html

2.   Reuters: CDC Director Redfield, "Facemasks are our best defence," September 2020

3.   'CDC calls on Americans to wear masks to prevent COVID-19 spread', JAMA editorial, Media Relations, July 2020 https://www.cdc.gov/media/releases/2020/p0714-americans-to-wear-masks.html

4.   E. O'Kelly et al. BMJ Open 2020, "Ability of fabric face mask materials to filter ultrafine at coughing velocity," Published September 2020, https://www.ncbi.nlm.nih.gov/pmc/articles/PMC7509966/

4.   Ibid; https://bmjopen.bmj.com/content/10/9/e039424

5.   Derek K Chu, MD et al. The Lancet, "Physical distancing, face masks, and eye protection to prevent person to person transmission of SARS- CoV-2 and COVID-19: systematic review and meta-analysis," June 2020;

172

https://www.thelancet.com/journals/lancet/article/PIIS0140-6736(20)31142-9/fulltext

6.   The Lancet, "Scientific consensus on the COVID-19 pandemic: we need to act now," October 2020; https://www.thelancet.com/journals/lancet/article/PIIS0140-6736(20)32153-X/fulltext

https://www.thelancet.com/journals/lancet

7.   Derek K Chu, MD et al. The Lancet, "Physical distancing, face masks, and eye protection to prevent person to person transmission of SARS- CoV-2 and COVID-19: systematic review and meta-analysis," June 2020; https://www.thelancet.com/journals/lancet/article/PIIS0140-6736(20)31142-9/fulltext

8.   Tom Jefferson, Carl Heneghan, "Masking lack of evidence with politics," July 2020, https://www.cebm.net/covid-19/masking-lack-of-evidence-with-politics/

9.   J. Howard et al, PNAS "An evidence review of face masks against COVID-19," January 2021; https://www.pnas.org/content/118/4/e2014564118

10.   C. Raina Macintyre et al, BMJ Open; "A cluster randomised trail of cloth masks compared with medical masks in healthcare workers,"

https://bmjopen.bmj.com/content/5/4/e006577

11.   CDC, Science Brief: "Community use of cloth masks to control the spread of Sars-CoV-2," May 2021, *https://www.cdc.gov/coronavirus/2019-ncov/science/science-briefs/masking-science-sars-cov2.html*.

12.   Lena H. Sun and Fenit Nirappil says, "Masks should fit better or be doubled up to protect against coronavirus variants CDC," February 2021; The Washing ton Post; *https://www.washingtonpost.com/health/2021/02/10/cdc-double-masks-covid/*

13.   BMJ Newsroom, "Time to encourage people to wear masks as a precaution says experts," April 2020, https://www.bmj.com/company/newsroom/time-to-encourage-people-to-wear-face-masks-as-a-precaution-say-experts/

14.   Irfan A. Dhalia, MD Msc and Joshua Tepper, MD MPH eMBA, "Improving the quality of healthcare in Canada," Oct. 2018; https://www.ncbi.nlm.nih.gov/pmc/articles/PMC6167219/

15.   'Reduction in OVID-19 Infection Using Surgical Facial Masks outside the Healthcare system', Clinical Trials. gov, US National Library of Medicine, April 2020, Updated August 2020; https://clinicaltrials.gov/ct2/show/NCT04337541

China Villain or victim...

1. Bruce Y. lee, Forbes, "Cases of COVID-19 jumped due to change in counting method," February 13, 2020, https://www.forbes.com/sites/brucelee/2020/02/13/new-coronavirus-covid-19-counting-method-leads-to-jump-in-cases-deaths/?sh=100eee7616af

2. Foreign & Commonwealth Office "Coronavirus outbreak: flights from China," February 2020, www.gov.uk/government/news/corona-virus-outbreak-flights-from-china

3. "Conspiracy Theory," Cambridge dictionary

4. Steve Strang, "God, Trump and COVID-19," 2020,

5. Celia Hatton BBC News, "China's Red Cross fights to win back trust," Beijing 22 April 2013 https://www.bbc.co.uk/news/world-asia-china-22244339

6. Ibid

7. Speech at the 40th Anniversary of the Publication of 'A letter to Compatriots in Taiwan', XI Jinping, January 2 2019

8. India Today "Controversial Wuhan P4 lab stayed open through Covid pandemic,"

https://www.indiatoday.in/world/story/controversial-wuhan-p4-lab-has-stayed-open-through-covid-pandemic-1709499-2020-08-09

9. The Changing Global Religious Landscape | Pew Research Center (pewforum.org), "The Changing Global Religious Landscape: Babies born to Muslims will begin to outnumber Christian births by 2035; people with no religion face a birth dearth," April 2017; https://www.pewforum.org/2015/04/02/religious-projections-2010-2050/

10. Ibid

11. Tom Cotton, Cotton Op-Ed in the Wall Street Journal, "Coronavirus and the laboratories in Wuhan," April 2020, https://www.cotton.senate.gov/news/press-releases/-cotton-op-ed-in-the-wall-street-journal-and-145coronavirus-and-the-laboratories-in-wuhan-and-146

12. 'Cotton Circumstantial Evidence Points Towards Wuhan Labs', John McCormack, National Review, April 22, 2020

13. Aiylin Woodward, Business Insider, "The new Corona virus has killed nearly 3 times as many people in 8 weeks as SARS, Did in 8 Months, Here' s How the 2 Outbreaks Compare," February 20, 2020,

14. Jane Parry, BMJ 329, no 7458 "Two Hong Kong Politicians Resign in the Wake of SARS," (July 17, 2004) 130,

15. Missionaries at border spread Christianity to North Korea, HYUNG-JIN KIM and GERRY SHIH April 5, 2018

16. Ibid

Chapter Three

Past, present and future

1.   Retro report By Clyde Haberman Oct 28, 2018, https://www.nytimes.com/2018/10/28/us/religion-politics-evangelicals.html.

In the last days

1.   Luke 21:10, 11
2.   Britannica Academic
3.   The Watchtower November 2, 2020.

Wind rush stories

1. The Guardian: I've been here for 50 years: the scandal of the former Commonwealth citizens threatened with deportation.

2. The Guardian: Windrush: two years on, victims describe long waits and 'abysmal' payouts

3. The Independent: Hundreds of Windrush victims still waiting as only 1 percent of compensation is paid

   The Independent: Nine out of ten Wind rush applicants still waiting for compensation payouts

4. The Independent: 'Hostile environment' broke law and is 'shameful stain on British history', equality watchdog finds

   The Guardian: Home Office broke equalities law with hostile environment measures

5. See note 4

6. 38 Degrees: Windrush: never again petition

7. The Guardian: Black official quit 'racist' Windrush compensation scheme

   The Independent: Black official quits 'racist' Windrush compensation scheme over its failure to help victims

Fighting the giant of fear...

1.   The Great Barrington Declaration, _https://www.politifact.com/factchecks/2020/oct/27/facebook-posts/great-barrington-herd-immunity-document-widely-dis/_

2.   Stephanie M. Lee, July 24, 2020, "An Elite Group of Scientists Tried to Warn Trump against Lockdowns in March"
https://www.buzzfeednews.com/article/stephaniemlee/ioannidis-trump-white-house-coronavirus-lockdowns

3.   Fear is killing us before the virus does...

4.   Prof Carl Heneghan claims: Data used to justify England's second national lockdown is 'proven' to be false,
https://www.telegraph.co.uk/news/2020/11/03/data-used-justify-englands-second-national-lockdown-proven-false/

5.   https://www.thebernician.net/treaty-of-universal-community-trust/

Immunity and immunization

1. Dr. Ronx Ikharia;   "The truth about .... BBC; boosting your immune system"

2. Ibid

3. Dr. Mohammed Shamgi,Imperial College London; "The truth about .... BBC; boosting your immune system."

4. Dr. Fluvio D'Aquuisto,Health Sciences Research Centre – University of Roehampton, UK; Use of massage in immunisation

5. Professor Michael Hienrich, 2021, UCL News, School of Pharmacy; "Which immune-boosting supplements work?"

6. Dr Ronx Ikharia, 2020, *BBC, The truth about...*

7.https://www.medrxiv.org/content/10.1101/2020.10.07.20208645v1

Chapter Four

Spirituality vs. Ego

1.   Chandresh Bhardwaj, Contributor, "Recognising and eliminating your spiritual ego," December 2017, https://www.huffpost.com/entry/recognizing-and-eliminati_b_5425001

2.   Psalms 91, NIV

3.   Southern Christian Leadership, Biography, January 1957, https://kinginstitute.stanford.edu/encyclopedia/southern-christian-leadership-conference-sclc

4.   Chris Parr, November 2016; https://www.timeshighereducation.com/blog/yesterday-i-wrote-about-trump-winning-election-i-never-thought-piece-would-be-published

5.   Just conversations with Kelly Brown Douglas / Tia Dole, Ph.D. July 2021;
  https://www.facebook.com/EDSatUnion/videos/36805926468542
  6

6.   Kelly Brown Douglas, Reflections, "Black Church Homophobia; what to do about it?" Spring 2006;
  https://reflections.yale.edu/article/sex-and-church

7.   I John 4:1

Chapter Five

I beg your pardon

1.   U.S.A. constitution Article 2

2.   https://sgp.fas.org/crs/misc/pardons.pdf

3.   Ibid

4.   The men who gave Trump his brutal world view, 2016;
  https://www.politico.com/magazine/story/2016/03/2016-donald-trump-brutal-worldview-father-coach-213750/

5.   Trump's right new right hand man has history of controversial clients, 2016;
  https://www.theguardian.com/us-news/2016/apr/27/paul-manafort-donald-trump-campaign-past-clients.

Notes

6.   'Political corruption', September 2019,
https://thehill.com/social-tags/political-corruption?page=1

7.   'Genome UK - the future of healthcare' (.PDF) -
GOV.UK

8.   Revelation 21:14, NKJV

9.   Mark 5:34, NKJV

10.   Psalm 103:1-5, NKJV

11.   Mathew 4:23, NKJV

12.   'CRISPR gene-editing treatment could reach
patients'very,very' soon', Intellia CEO, published July 2021,
https://www.cnbc.com/2021/07/02/crispr-gene-editing-could-
reach-patients-very-soon-intellia-ceo.html

13.   'Appications of gene-editing technology I targeted
therapy of human diseases...'
https://www.nature.com/articles/s41392-019-0089-y

14.   'The cost of sequencing the human genome', National
Human Genome Reseach Institute,
https://www.genome.gov/about-genomics/fact-
sheets/Sequencing-Human-Genome-cost

15.   The Great Barrington Declaration

16.   Wikipedia

17.   Laura Romero et al, 2020,Kizzmekia Corbett .an African American is praised as key scientist behind COVID -19 vaccine;
https://abcnews.go.com/Health/kizzmekia-corbett-african-american-woman-praised-key-scientist/story?id=74679965

18.   Analysis of the Tuskegee experiment, 2004
https://www.bartleby.com/essay/Analysis-Of-The-Tuskegee-Experiment-P35T74TYS4FF

19.   'The Washington Post, Can the 'immortal cells' of Henrietta Lacks sue for their own rights?' De Neen L. Brown, 2018,
https://www.washingtonpost.com/news/retropolis/wp/2018/06/25

20.   'Kizzmekia Corbett an African American is praised as key scientist behind COVID -19 vaccine,' Laura Romero et al, 2020,
https://abcnews.go.com/Health/kizzmekia-corbett-african-american-woman-praised-key-scientist/story?id=74679965

21.   Meet the black female scientist at the fore front of COVID-19 vaccine development, Jan 2021,

https://www.cbsnews.com/news/covid-19-vaccine-development-kizzmekia-corbett/

22.   COVID-19 vaccines and people of colour, John Hopkins medicine;
https://www.hopkinsmedicine.org/health/conditions-and-diseases/coronavirus/covid19-vaccines-and-people-of-color

23.   'UK aims to give first COVID-19 vaccine by; September', Danica Kirka, January 2021;
https://apnews.com/article/business-coronavirus-pandemic-coronavirus-vaccine-89797ad678c18042d18386985a38859e

24.   News, May 2021,
https://www.nature.com/articles/d41586-020-00502-w

25.   'COVID-19:vaccine success means we have to look at data differently', Ed Conway, June 2021,
https://news.sky.com/story/covid-19-the-vaccines-success-means-we-have-to-look-at-the-data-differently-12341925

Chapter Six

Who is responsible...

1.   Boris Johnson faces questions over death toll,
https://www.theguardian.com/world/2021/jan/26/ons-figures-show-uk-passed-100000-covid-deaths-by-7-january

2.   Reuters," *U.K. Opposition Leader Denounces Boris Johnson Handling of Corona Crisis,"* September 22, 2020,

3.   Reuters, "Mass cremations begin as India's capital faces deluge Covid - 19 deaths," 22 April 2021,
https://www.reuters.com/world/india/mass-cremations-begin-indias-capital-faces-deluge-covid-19-deaths-2021-04-23/

4.   Office of National Statistics (ONS) *"Deaths registered weekly in England and Wales, provisional: week ending 3 April 2020."*

5.   "U.K. virus deaths exceed 100,000 since pandemic began"
https://www.bbc.co.uk/news/health-55757378

6.   LBC.co.uk, *report, "More than 400 daily care home deaths at peak of UK Covid outbreak,"* Sept 4, 2020;

7.   The King's Fund, Veena Raleigh, *"Deaths from COVID-19 (coronavirus): how are they counted and what do they show?"* 23 April 2021,

8.   Press release: Kate Bingham appointed new chair of UK vaccine taskforce, May 16, 2020;
https://www.gov.uk/government/news/kate-bingham-appointed-chair-of-uk-vaccine-taskforce

Managing Grief

1. Lianna Champ, *"How to Grieve Like A Cham,"* June 2018;

Notes

2. Elisabeth Kübler-Ross, "Five stages of grief," 1969;

What would I do better...

1. Chistainhelpfordepression.org

2. Champ, "15 Ideas for Bereavement Gifts That Show You Care," Https://champfunerals.com/ideas-for-bereavement-gifts/

3. Ibid

4. Ibid

5. Philippians 2:4 NKJV Bible;

6. https://liberalamerica.org/2015/11/17/what-does-the-bible-say-about-helping-your-fellow-man-for-example-refugees/

Afterword

1. Alice Palmer, Mailonline, "Lewis Hamilton's Latest Business Venture Sparks Tension With Big Pharma - He Fires Back Live On Air!" August 21, 2021.

2. https://www.itv.com/news/2021-09-02/coronavirus-vaccination-halves-risk-of-long-covid

3. Ibid

4. Professor Tim Spector - UK Zoe COVID Symptom Study,

- Clyde Haberman Oct 28,2018
- See for instance the following selections: Jerry Bergman, Journal of Creation 13, no.1 "Did God Make Pathogenic Viruses?" (1999):115–125, https://answersingenesis.org/who-is-god/god-is-good/did-god-make-pathogenic-viruses/
- Andrew Fabich, "Celebrate Your Inner Virus," Answers in Depth 12 (2017), https://answersingenesis.org/biology/microbiology/celebrate-your-inner-virus/
- Andrew Fabich, "Where Did Ebola Come From?" Answers in Depth 9 (2014), https://answersingenesis.org/biology/microbiology/where-did-ebola-come-from/;
- Andrew Fabich, "The Flu: Everything You Need to Know," Answers in Depth 12 (2017), https://answersingenesis.org/biology/disease/flu-everything-you-need-to-know/;

Notes

o Andrew Fabich, "The Beneficial Functions of Endogenous Retroviruses," Answers in Depth 11 (2016), https://answersingenesis.org/biology/microbiology/beneficial-functions-endogenous-retroviruses/;

o Joe Francis, "The Organosubstrate of Life," Answers in Depth 4 (2009), https://answersingenesis.org/biology/microbiology/the-organosubstrate-of-life/

o Luke Kim, "Bacterial Attenuation and its Link to Innate Oncolytic Potential," Answers Research Journal 1 (2008), https://answersingenesis.org/natural-selection/antibiotic-resistance/bacterial-attenuation-and-its-link-to-innate-oncolytic-potential/;

o Ryan Lucas Kitner, "Genetic Variance of Influenza Type A Avian Virus and its Evolutionary Implications," Answers in Depth 1 (2006), https://answersingenesis.org/natural-selection/antibiotic-resistance/influenza-type-a-and-its-evolutionary-implications/;

o Yingguang Liu, "Cyclic Selection in HIV-1 Tropism: Microevolution That is Going Nowhere," Answers Research Journal 8 (2018):199–202, https://answersingenesis.org/biology/disease/cyclic-selection-hiv-1-tropism/;

o Yingguang Liu, "Mutations in the nef Gene make HIV-1 More Virulent," Answers Research Journal 8 (2018):323–326. https://answersingenesis.org/biology/disease/mutations-in-nef-gene-make-hiv-1-more-virulent/;

o Yingguang Liu, "Is HIV-1 Losing Fitness Due to Genetic Entropy?" Answers Research Journal 8 (2018):339–351, https://answersingenesis.org/biology/disease/is-hiv-1-losing-fitness-due-to-genetic-entropy/;

o Yingguang Liu and Charles Soper, "The Natural History of Retroviruses," Answers Research Journal 2 (2009):97–106, https://answersingenesis.org/genetics/the-natural-history-of-retroviruses/

o Elizabeth Mitchell, "Endogenous Retroviruses: Key to Mammalian Brain Development?" Answers in Depth 10 (2015), https://answersingenesis.org/biology/microbiology/endogenous-retroviruses-key-to-mammalian-brain-development/;

o Jean O'Micks, "Creation perspective of nucleocytoplasmic large DNA viruses." Journal of Creation 30, no. 3 (2016):110–117;

Warren A. Shipton, Journal of Creation 30, no. 2 "Origins of pathogenic microbes: part 2-viruses," (2016): 78–87.

Printed in Great Britain
by Amazon

21054162R00119